Doin' the Locum Motion

Doin' the Locum Motion

Chris Rolton

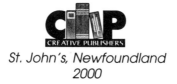
CREATIVE PUBLISHERS

St. John's, Newfoundland
2000

Le Conseil des Arts | The Canada Council
du Canada | for the Arts

We acknowledge the support of The Canada Council for the Arts for
our publishing program.

We acknowledge the financial support of the Government of Canada
through the Book Publishing Industry Development Program (BPDIP)
for our publishing activities.

Cover art: Robin LeDrew

∞ Printed on acid-free paper

Published by

CREATIVE BOOK PUBLISHING
a division of 10366 Newfoundland Limited
a Robinson-Blackmore Printing & Publishing associated company
P.O. Box 8660, St. John's, Newfoundland A1B 3T7

First Edition

Printed in Canada by:
ROBINSON-BLACKMORE PRINTING & PUBLISHING

Canadian Cataloguing in Publication Data

Rolton, Chris, 1939-

Doin' the locum motion ·

ISBN 1-894294-26-2

1. Rolton, Chris, 1939-
2. Substitute physicians — Canada, Northern — Biography.   I. Title

R729.5.R87R64   2000   610'.92   C00-950163-0

Dedication

Table of Contents

Part 4:Back To Newfoundland

Credits for previously published sections of this book:

"American Visitors" was originally published in *The Medical Post* on 3.3.87 as "What? Our New Doctor's a She?"

"Two Pioneers" was originally published (in a slightly different form) in *The Medical Post* on 5 Aug 86 as "Albert and Alice were the last of their kind."

A portion of "Two Rescues" was originally published in *Family Practice* on 30.1.90 as "A Winter Fire at a Lonely Fishing Camp."

"Gaston" was originally published in *The Medical Post* on 21.3.89 as "Alcohol Abuse: It became one miner's major problem"

"Cottage Country Weekend" was originally published in *The Medical Post* on 1 April 86 as "A Quiet Summer in Cottage Country" and 22 April 86 as "A Shift in Cottage Country No Picnic."

"House Calls" was originally published in The Medical Post on 19.9.89 as "Finding the Patient's House is Nine-Tenths of the Battle when you're a Rural Locum."

"It's How We Say It" was originally published in *The Medical Post* on 22.5.90 as "I Feels Right Logy, Doc"

"Doctor as Vet" was originally published in *The Medical Post* on 23.8.88 as "It sounds catty but I'm a doggy doctor from Labrador."

"A Vicious Attack" was originally published in *Family Practice* in Fall 90 as "A Vicious Attack and a Slow Recovery."

"It's a Disaster!" was originally published in *The Medical Post* on 20 March 90 as "Mock Emergencies can easily turn into Real Disasters."

Foreword

For over twenty years I substituted for sick and vacationing doctors in various parts of Canada; mostly in rural, sometimes remote, areas, where the work is so much more interesting and worthwhile than city medicine.

After two years in Labrador I headed west. Finally, I returned east to settle on the island of Newfoundland, my home for many years now.

All the incidents described really happened, but have been rearranged to make stories. The people and places are real, but disguised and renamed to protect them (and me). Except for the late Dr. Tony Paddon who, after a lifetime of medical service, became Lieutenant-Governor of Newfoundland and Labrador. Respected, loved and liked, he needs no camouflage.

—Chris Rolton 1998

Part 1: Labrador

A New Life

From the plane window the country looked flat and dull. Between the numerous pewter-grey lakes, areas of dark green, interspersed with patches of brown and white, passed by below. I was arriving at Gander for the first time, after traveling all day, first to Heathrow, then across the Atlantic. It was 23 November 1967, the real beginning of my life. Tomorrow, I would journey on to Labrador. The very name sounded remote and challenging. This would surely be different from English suburbia!

We landed. I struggled into my coat and off the plane. There was no room in my luggage for the heavy winter coat and boots I had been advised to purchase, so I was wearing them, and found them hot and cumbersome. Crossing the tarmac to the terminal, I took a quick look round. The grey clouds glowered at the flat brown landscape. The wind was icy and even the trees looked cold.

The balding, middle-aged Immigration Officer checked my papers and passport.

"Where are you going from here?" he questioned me.

"Goose Bay."

"Goose Bay! What are you going there for?"

"I've got a job there. Why? What's wrong with the place?"

"It's a bit isolated for a young lady like you to go to."

"Aren't there any young men there?" I asked, mischievously.

"I dare say. Americans mostly. They have a base there."

This really surprised me. I was expecting Indians and Eskimos, not Americans. He returned my documents and waved me on.

"Good luck."

Picking up my luggage I crossed to the EPA desk to confirm my flight for the next day.

"You can't go to Goose Bay tomorrow," the young clerk told me, "there aren't no flights."

"But I've got a ticket," I cried, producing it.

"I'll put you on for the next day, if there's a seat. Yes, that should be OK."

He adjusted my ticket and turned to his next customer.

Tired and a bit discouraged, I took a taxi to the Holiday Inn. They, at least, were expecting me, and I was soon checked in and shown to my room. I had never stayed in a hotel before, and was dazzled by its opulence and warmth. Used to British cold, damp houses, and piles of blankets on the beds, I was amazed to sit comfortably in shirt sleeves.

Next morning after breakfast I tried to call the hospital in Goose Bay, to inform them of my delay, but couldn't get through.

"Likely the circuits is busy," said the pretty young desk clerk helpfully.

1 wandered out for a walk, wondering what I would do all day. I was itching to get to Labrador, and Gander seemed so dreary. At a store I bought a couple of chocolate bars, and a book of crossword puzzles. When it started to rain I returned to the hotel. This time I got through to Goose Bay and advised them of the hitch. They were very nonchalant about it. When I knew EPA better I understood why.

Ten minutes later I was enjoying a coffee in the restaurant when the desk clerk came running in.

"Was you wanting to go to Goose Bay today? They's leaving in twenty minutes. Shall I call you a taxi?"

Completely astonished, I flew up to my room, packed up, and raced down to the lobby and into a taxi. At the airport I was taken to a back room meant only for the crew. A rather scruffy middle-aged man sat there, smoking and reading a newspaper.

"No hurry," he said, comfortably, "we're not ready yet."

"How come there's a flight today after all?" I asked.

"Plane that's up there's broken down, so I've got to take another one down."

"Are you the pilot?"

"Sure."

He stubbed out his cigarette, gave me the paper, and sauntered out along the corridor. I helped myself to a cup of awful coffee from the urn in the corner, read the paper — the previous day's — then sat staring out the window. The skies had cleared and the sun shone brightly. A plane stood just outside, waiting hopefully, a black and white cat curled up asleep in a puddle of sun by one of the wheels.

The pilot reappeared, picked up my luggage, and jerked his head for me to follow him. We climbed aboard, and he tucked my luggage in by the front seats. Waving his arm to indicate the whole empty plane, he offered,

"Take a seat, any one you like."

For the first half hour or so I watched the coast go by, as we flew down the eastern side of the Great Northern Peninsula. The green and brown hills set off the vivid glittering blue of the sea. Tiny scattered outports clung at the edge, looking very isolated, as indeed they were. We crossed the Strait of Belle Isle over to Labrador. Now the land was mostly white, and there were no houses at all. It looked cold, harsh and desolate.

Two hours from Gander we landed at Goose Bay. As we walked to the shed that was the terminal in those days, the pilot kindly carrying my suitcases, I suddenly realized that the hospital was not expecting me until the next day. How far away was it? How would I get there? From the runway I could

see nothing but flat snow and a few, obviously military buildings. There were no taxis in sight, and I wasn't then used to
the way one can use other people's phones so readily here. At
the counter the clerk suggested I call them and get someone
to come and pick me up. Unaware that the hospital had a
truck for various errands, including conveying people to and
from the airport, I hesitated.

Then the clerk told me to hold on a minute; that Mountie
was likely going to the hospital. He waved energetically to a
man outside. He came in and I saw my first real Mountie. It
was a big disappointment. Aside from his furry hat, he was
just like any other policeman. No scarlet tunic and Boy Scout
hat. He was young and appeared in the best of health, and I
wondered why the clerk thought he was going to the hospital.
The Mountie very willingly offered me a ride and I, and my
bags, were soon stowed in his car. We chatted pleasantly and
discussed my journey. Apparently the mixup over the flights,
the frantic call to be at the airport in twenty minutes, then the
two hour wait, were "EPA all over." As we turned off the road
I saw the RCMP headquarters to my right, and the hospital to
my left — explaining the airport clerk's seeming clairvoy-
ance. The Mountie took me to the administrator's office.

"Hi Buddy. This is your new doctor. EPA got her all
fooled up, but here she is."

The administrator, who really was known as Buddy, took
his feet off his desk and put them on the floor, stubbed out his
cigarette and shook my hand.

"You must have had a long day. Come and have a cup of
tea."

As I had had nothing since breakfast, except for the coffee
at Gander, and the two chocolate bars, long since gone, I was
starving. Gratefully, I followed him to the staff lounge.

Settling In

For the first few weeks I was hypnotized by the huge snow-covered spaces, great stands of spruce trees, and colourful wooden houses, all sparkling in the sunshine. As I had expected the patients were Innu (Indian), Inuit (Eskimo) and white, all living their rugged lives in tune with their environment. Most of my colleagues were from away, several being British.

But the Director was born and raised in Labrador and, apart from his time at medical school and in the Navy, had lived his whole life there. Dr. Tony Paddon was a remarkable man. His skills in a wide variety of medical problems, his knowledge of the land and the people, and his kindly tolerance of us brash know-it-alls from across the Atlantic, made him a unique boss. His delightful sense of humour and quick wit defused many stressful situations.

One evening, soon after I arrived and was just beginning to find my way around, I walked to the door with him as he departed for his home. Almost immediately he returned and beckoned to me.

"You seen the northern lights yet? They don't come any better than this."

I followed him outside in my sandals. A great shimmering purple, green and white curtain undulated across the sky, filling it from horizon to horizon. Awestruck, I stared and stared, unable to find anything to say.

"Go back inside or you'll freeze," advised Dr Paddon, bringing me back to earth with a bump, "And don't expect much from the radio tomorrow. The reception will be awful."

Living always in the south of England I had never known a white Christmas. Indeed I had very little experience of snow at all. On December 23, when I had been in Labrador a month, the hospital held its staff party.

Snow was falling softly, and the view from the window was as "Christmassy" as one could wish. As I watched, two men pulling komatiks (sleds) each laden with three or four trees, emerged from the woods and tramped by on their way to their homes. It seemed incredible to me, used to paying at least two pounds (four dollars) for a pathetic little tree for the living room, that here one could go out and select the best — free. Only the day before Tom, a hospital maintenance man/ ambulance driver, had cut four — three for the hospital and one for his home.

A jingle of bells, and a hearty "Ho! Ho! Ho!" drew me back to the celebrations. Santa had arrived. Bert, the other maintenance man/ ambulance driver made a natural Santa. Burly and bearded, he joked and chatted as he passed out the gifts from his sack. When the party, with its laughter and carol-singing, was over, the five-year-old son of one of the other doctors came up to me, his blue eyes shining ecstatically.

"I always wondered what Santa did all year. Now I know. He works here!"

Next day the sun shone again, but the temperature dropped to minus twenty-five. As I walked the short distance to the Anglican church for the midnight service, the snow squeaking under my boots and the northern lights dancing about the sky, I recalled my last Christmas in a gloomy industrial town in England. Though mild, it had been very wet and depressing. It hardly seemed possible that I was on the same planet.

On New Year's Eve several of us — another doctor, two teachers, a nurse, a lab technician and me — went icefishing on the river. The sunshine dazzled on the snow, but the wind was bitter. Strolling around in my new mukluks (sealskin boots) and new "Grenfell" parka I snapped photographs of the others chopping holes in the ice, then squatting down to fish through them. Trying to get a better picture, and completely ignorant about river ice, I thoughtlessly walked further out than I should have.

Suddenly, there was a creak and a crash and I was up to my neck in icy water.

"Don't run anybody or we'll all be in," shouted a male voice, "I'll go and get help."

Kicking my legs furiously I tried to grab onto the ice. The first time it broke away. The same thing happened the second time. But the third time it held, and I was able to haul my elbows up onto it. Assisted by encouraging yells from my friends, and still kicking like mad, I somehow heaved myself out and crawled towards them. They yanked me to my feet and half carried, half pushed me to the bank, where a skidoo was just pulling up. The teacher had run to the nearest house where, fortunately, the owner was not only home but had a skidoo, and came immediately.

I sat on behind and in five minutes was at the hospital door. But the water in my clothes had frozen, and I couldn't straighten out. The poor man had to practically carry me into the hospital lobby, where he sat me on the nearest chair and went for a nurse. It was warm there, and by the time he returned, I was starting to drip.

Upstairs in the staff quarters I soon stripped and dried off. It wasn't until I was drinking a hot cup of tea that I started to shiver, with shock and fright rather than cold. The rest of the party had returned, and walked me up and down the corridor to get my circulation going, before letting me curl up in an armchair and relax.

That evening my legs became painful, and very tender to touch. Putting on pantyhose for the Hogmanay party at the dentist's, I found that I couldn't bear even that very slight pressure, so I changed into socks and smooth slacks. Hardly able to walk, I slithered across to the house nearby hanging on to two stalwart nurses. When I sat down the feel of the slacks against my legs was almost intolerable. Once midnight had passed I returned to the hospital and crawled into bed. With the weight of the bedclothes on my tender legs I didn't sleep that well.

Next morning my legs were one huge black and blue bruise. There was no question of getting into pantyhose or slacks, and I spent the day (luckily a Sunday) in my housecoat. Dr Paddon came over after church (informed, I later discovered, by a nurse at the same service) and was very concerned and kind. He explained about ruptured capillaries and cold antibodies, then sternly pointed out that the current was very fast there. I was lucky, he said, not to be pulled under and "gone for good."

Over the next week my bruises subsided, and I could dress normally again. The episode caused quite a stir in the community, and patients invariably inquired,

"Was it you fell in the river, miss?"

Months later Ralph, the pilot of our bushplane/ambulance, handed me a camera.

"That yours?" he asked.

It was. A fisherman, way down at Rigolet, had caught it in his net and given it to Ralph, who guessed I had dropped it when the ice gave way. That film, of course, was ruined. But I tried a new one and the pictures were fine. That cheap little camera did many years service.

Death and Alcohol

Two weeks later, when I had recovered from my fright and was fully mobile again, I had another lesson in respect for the severe winter weather. One morning, as I was preparing for the prenatal clinic, Dr Paddon came into the room, accompanied by a Mountie.

"Chris, could you go with Constable Lipinsky to look at a body?" said Dr Paddon. "Just pronounce him dead, and they'll bring him here for autopsy. If he's thawed out enough we'll do it this afternoon. If not, tomorrow morning."

I checked the two patients already waiting, hung the "BACK SOON" notice on the clinic door, and joined the Mountie for my second skidoo ride.

The snow-laden spruce trees towered on each side of the narrow trail, leaving just a streak of deep blue sky above. In five minutes he drew up beside another Mountie and cut the engine. The silence was profound. Nothing stirred as I stood listening.

"He's right here, Doc. Come and have a look, then I'll run you back to the hospital."

The man lay on his left side, his right hand on a large gun. An erratic trail of blood spots led right up to him.

"Did he shoot himself?" I asked.

"No. He got drunk and had an argument with another drunk, and they shot at each other. This guy missed his mark altogether, but caught one himself."

"Where's the wound?"

Constable Lipinsky bent down to show me. To my surprise it was in the calf of the man's leg.

"He died of that?" I queried, puzzled. "There's not much blood."

"No, no, Doc. He fell down and froze to death, I'd say. Dr Paddon will tell us for sure when he does the autopsy."

"What about the other fellow?"

"He was sleeping it off when we called. Really upset, he is."

"What will he be charged with? Manslaughter?" I wondered, aloud.

"Assault causing grievous bodily harm, maybe. Careless use of a firearm, probably. They were friends, and he obviously didn't intend to kill him."

"But why were they carrying their guns?"

He shrugged, then grinned. "You a lawyer as well as a doctor?"

"No. I guess I'd better get back to the clinic."

Next morning Dr Paddon did the autopsy while Constable Lipinsky and I made notes on his findings. As he worked Dr Paddon told us how one of his fall chores, along with raking the leaves and covering his rose bushes, was "guestimating" the deaths in the coming winter and getting the graves dug, as this was impossible once the cold weather set in. He sighed.

"There should be plenty left this early, though I didn't include him in my calculations. He was only thirty-five and has a young family. What a waste! A basically decent, honest fellow dying quite unnecessarily."

"The other man is really, really upset," said Constable Lipinsky. And it's not just because he'll go to prison either, I don't think."

"You got him in the lockup at Goose Bay?" asked Dr Paddon.

The Mountie nodded.

"I'll drop in and see him when I'm over there tomorrow," continued Dr Paddon. "He'll bear this burden the rest of his life."

"What if you guess wrong and don't have enough graves?" I asked.

"We put them in the shed until the ground thaws out. They don't rot at all in these temperatures."

By now, he had confirmed that death was primarily due to exposure, aggravated by alcohol and a bullet wound in the leg.

Next day I went to Goose Bay with Dr Paddon in his posh new Pontiac to do some shopping. Halfway there he pulled up, and turned to me with a smile.

"You want to drive this thing for a bit?"

I was astounded, but changed places with him eagerly. Having only driven an old Mini, I could hardly believe how easily the huge car flew along. The lightest touch on the wheel and accelerator and we zoomed up hills and around corners, the trees whizzing by. A rabbit hopping across the road caused me to brake, and the car stopped so suddenly it almost went into spin.

"Gently now," cautioned Dr Paddon, "Next rabbit you see clip it, and I'll take it home for supper."

We drove on, but the rabbits had been warned and kept out of our way. As I turned into the hospital parking lot Buddy, the administrator, was standing on the back steps chatting with the Catholic priest. I swept past them and pulled into the parking area just beyond, again stopping rather suddenly. When he saw me at the wheel Buddy's jaw dropped. Dr Paddon and the priest greeted each other and entered the hospital, followed by Buddy and me.

"He let you drive his brand new car!" exclaimed Buddy in amazement. I nodded; only then did it occur to me that Dr Paddon had never even asked me if I could drive.

On the way home I asked him if he had visited the man in the lockup.

"Yes. He's really down, as you'd expect. Clearly it was an accident, and completely out of character. But he'll have to pay for it. I imagine the Judge will be as lenient as he can with the jail sentence. He'll know that it will be on the man's conscience for ever. It's all very sad."

He pulled over and got out of the car.

"Be back in a minute," he called, and headed for the trees. Thinking he had gone for a "leak" I was surprised to see him pick up a small rock. He threw it up into the nearest tree then plodded over, picked something up off the ground and brought it back to the car. He showed me a large bird, then put it in the trunk.

As we headed off again, he said, "Spruce grouse are so dumb! They just sit there and let you take them like that. I'll pluck it later and we'll have it for supper tomorrow."

"Then what would you have done with the rabbit, if I'd hit it?"

"Oh, they keep well for days in this cold. We'd have had it next day."

Several evenings later Dr Paddon was at the hospital, seeing a seriously ill child, when the snowplow driver rushed in.

"Dr Paddon! Dr Paddon! I knocked someone down! I think he was drunk. He staggered right in front of me. I didn't have time to stop."

Shuddering, he sat down suddenly on a nearby chair, and buried his face in his hands.

"Did you see who it was?" asked Dr Paddon in his gentle way.

The driver named him.

"Then, more than likely he was drunk," continued Dr Paddon, quietly. "It was his usual condition. Where is he?"

He followed the driver out into the blizzard and returned a few minutes later looking rather pale.

"Good job Leonard did recognize him," he said. "He's, well, pulverized, I suppose you'd call it."

Taking the janitor, a large plastic sheet and two shovels he went back outside. Later, he broke the news to the widow, home with their four small children, the youngest only a month old.

"Perhaps it's for the best," he remarked next morning. "He's always been a drunken ne'er-do-well. Now at least there'll be money for food and heat, and she won't get beaten up anymore."

He wrote up the death certificate — "multiple injuries incompatible with life" — and mailed it to St. John's. A month later it was returned, with a note requesting him to "be more specific."

"What do they want me to say?" he cried, in a rare burst of annoyance. "That he used to be five feet six inches tall and twelve inches thick, and became eight feet tall and half an inch thick?"

After some thought, he wrote, "crushed chest and fractured skull, with severe brain damage," and returned the death certificate.

Two Pioneers

One fine morning Craig Barnes, the young United Church minister, called me at the hospital.

"Chris? I'm going to visit the Andersons this afternoon. Want to come?"

"I'd love to! But I have a clinic to do. We can't all go joyriding in the middle of a workday, you know."

"This is a pastoral visit. I'll take communion to them, and some magazines I have here. Do they need any medications I could deliver for you?"

"They neither of them take anything, but thanks. You know their son, Warren, broke his ankle slipping on the ice outside the Hudson Bay Company?"

"Yes, that's partly why I'm going now. He won't be on a skidoo for a week or two, I guess."

"Right. Have a good trip."

After we hung up I returned to my paperwork, but just sat there at the desk remembering my visit to the Andersons a few weeks earlier.

. . .

That too had been a sparkling day of brilliant sunshine, without a whisper of wind. Then the stillness was broken by an explosion of noise as Craig started the skidoo. I climbed on behind and we roared down the narrow trail between the trees. Suddenly, the country opened out onto a large expanse of dazzling snow, untouched except for animal tracks a few feet away. Craig stopped the skidoo and turned off the engine. The silence was deafening. Nothing stirred.

"Those look like wolf tracks," commented Craig, adding, "In summer this is a swamp. Too boggy to walk in, but not wet enough for a boat. And insects! They love it here. To get to the Andersons then you have to go a long way round, either through the woods, or round the coast by boat. Like many places here, it's more accessible in the winter, when everything is frozen. Have you met the Andersons before?"

"No, but I've heard about them. They're Warren's parents, aren't they?"

"Yes. They must be way up on their eighties. After all, Warren is fifty and is, I believe, the youngest of their surviving children."

"Did they lose some then?"

"There are two tiny graves by the cabin. You won't see them today. They'll be under snow."

"It must have been a hard life. What did they do? Fish? Trap?"

"Oh yes, Albert was an expert trapper. Each spring he brought his furs to the Bay by sled. They were always top quality. Then he'd load up the sled with supplies and walk home again. Sometimes, Alice and the family went too. In the summer they had a garden, and fished. Very self-sufficient they were. We'd better get on."

He started the skidoo and jumped on and we were on our way. Twenty minutes later we pulled up at a small cabin in a clearing. Tall spruce trees grew around three sides, looming over yet sheltering the tiny dwelling. On the fourth side a small lake glittered with ice. At a hole near the shore, a man, bulky in his heavy clothing, was hauling out a sizable fish, still flapping a little. He laid it gently on the ice and waddled towards us.

"Come in, come in out of the cold both of you," a gentle voice urged beside us; and there was Alice, tiny and white-haired, with bright brown eyes and a delightful smile. "Welcome, Reverend. It is good of you to come all this way."

I was introduced.

"This is very kind of you, Doctor, but we're both perfectly well you know."

"I came for the trip," I told her. "I haven't even brought my stethoscope. This is a beautiful spot, and so quiet."

"We love it here. The town is so noisy, and people everywhere! I suppose we've got used to it here."

"After sixty-five years I guess we have."

I turned, to see Albert closing the door behind him. Not a big or fat man, now that he had shed his boots and parka. He shook hands.

"We're not sick, Doctor, but it's kind of you to come. Did you bring the Communion things, Reverend?" he asked Craig.

"Sure, I'll get ready."

"We aren't fasting," said Alice anxiously. "In fact, we had a big dinner. Albert snared a rabbit yesterday. It was tasty."

"You don't have to be fasting. Don't worry about it," said Craig cheerfully.

"Years ago," reminisced Albert, settling himself on the chesterfield by the woodstove, "We had a minister who was most particular about it. Big, fat feller he was. Didn't look as if he fasted much, I can tell you. Fasting is for those who've run out of food, as far as I can see. Plenty of that when we were young. You from England?"

I nodded.

"My ancestors came from Devon and Alice's from Somerset. You from there?"

"No, I'm from Sussex, but I've visited Devon and Somerset. It's nice country still, and not as full of people as Sussex."

Alice joined him on the chesterfield and I took the remaining easy chair, also covered with a colourful crocheted rug. While Craig conducted the short service I sat back comfortably, enjoying the smell of the woodstove and looking about the small room.

On the other side of the stove from the chesterfield stood the kitchen table and chairs, in front of cupboards built into the wall. A rack of fearsome-looking knives was nailed to the adjacent wall; a basket of vegetables hung from the ceiling on a large hook.

Behind the chesterfield, where the old couple sat quietly accepting the wafers and wine, a double bed was built into the corner. At its foot sat a small chest of drawers: two hairbrushes and a jar of "Vaseline" were arranged neatly to one side, a shaving mirror, brush and razor to the other. As Alice got up to make tea, I noticed a trapdoor in the ceiling.

"When the youngsters were growing up they slept up there," explained Albert. "We had a ladder for them. Until they could climb the ladder they stayed down here with us. You met Warren? He's our youngest."

"Yes, I've met him. He's the janitor at the school isn't he? Do your other children live around here?"

"Two of them have a fishing camp over at Beaver Creek. We don't see much of any of them except Warren, but they're doing all right. Some have children, and even grandchildren, now. We're getting old."

Craig and I enjoyed tea and homemade cookies, then left. Our visit was much appreciated, but they were obviously content to be by themselves again.

As I was finishing the clinic, and awaiting the results of bloodwork on a Mountie I suspected of having hepatitis, I heard a commotion at the Emergency entrance and went to investigate.

Maria, a tiny nurse from the Philippines (and often mistaken for an Inuk) was trying to manipulate a cumbersome stretcher out through the door. One wheel was sticking in an awkward position and the stretcher wouldn't go straight. A patient with his arm in a sling was trying to help her. A skidoo was parked just outside. Craig was bending over supporting his passenger and calling to Maria to hurry.

"I can't find a wheelchair," panted Maria. "That's why I'm trying to get this stretcher out there."

We shoved it through the doorway and alongside the skidoo, where Albert Anderson, purple and sweating, gasped for breath and clung to Craig.

"Come on!" urged Craig impatiently. "Can't you see he's all in? He's really sick."

Craig, Maria and I heaved Albert onto the stretcher between us; we raised the head end so that he could lean back against it. In the Emergency Room, Maria hooked him up to some oxygen while Craig and I wrestled his parka off.

"It's old Uncle Albert, isn't it?" asked the man with the sling. "He don't look too good, do he? Can I help?"

"You could go and find Dr.Paddon," I said. "He's probably in his office. What happened, Craig?"

"Late last night he brought the firewood in. Then he went out again and shovelled a bucketful of snow and brought it in to melt for the morning. That was when he got a pain in his chest and turned weak. Alice helped him to bed and the pain eased up. But since then he's found it difficult to breathe and has been sick to his stomach. Coughed a few times too."

"Of course, they've got no electricity, let alone a phone," Craig continued. "When I got there Alice was sitting with him and trying to get him to drink a cup of tea. She looked wiped out. Guess she'd been up all night. It wasn't easy to persuade him to come in. He was quite satisfied to stay there and die. I hope I did the right thing."

"I don't see what else you could have done," I said. "Could you find Warren and get him over here?"

"Sure," agreed Craig and left.

Albert had obviously had a heart attack and was now in heart failure. Dr. Paddon and I put up an intravenous and gave him some medication. Soon he was looking much better and lay back gratefully. For a few minutes he dozed quietly. Dr. Paddon looked across the stretcher at me and shook his head slightly, indicating that he thought Albert was not going to live.

Maria returned from Medical Records.

"I can't find an old chart on him, or even his card number."

"I doubt he's been here before," said Dr.Paddon. "Certainly I don't remember either of them ever needing us."

Warren Anderson, brought by Craig, hobbled in on crutches. His father opened his eyes and peered up at him.

"Hi Pa. How ye doing?"

"No good, no good. Your Ma. There by herself. No good."

"Don't worry, Pa. I'll get David to go tomorrow. It's getting too dark now. He's a favourite with his nan and he'll get her to come back with him; she'll want to see you."

His father nodded and drifted off again. Dr. Paddon beckoned to Warren and took him to the waiting room to talk to him while Maria and I got the old man upstairs to the ward.

An hour later, while I was at supper, the nurse on duty went to check him again, and found him dead.

Next morning Craig set out, again in brilliant sunshine, to inform Alice of Albert's death and arrange his funeral. By noon, he was back, with Alice riding pillion behind him. Pulling up at the Emergency entrance, he helped her off the skidoo and led her gently inside. Seeing my office door open, he brought her right over.

"Chris, Alice has burnt her hand. It looks nasty to me and must be painful."

I glanced at her, pale and drawn, but alert and upright.

"I'm sorry about Albert," I said. "But there wasn't any more we could do, you know."

She shook her head.

"He was eighty-nine, Doctor, and had never been ill in his life. I'm so thankful he didn't suffer for long."

Her eyes glistened suddenly and she gave me a small smile.

"He was always so busy! If he had lived and not been able to do much it would have driven him crazy! He wouldn't have wanted that."

Maria came to the door and was introduced to Alice by Craig.

"Can you take her to the treatment room and I'll come and look at her?" I asked Maria as my phone rang.

Two minutes later I was examining Alice's raw and blistered wrist. I asked her what happened.

"I was lifting that big kettle off the stove and dropped it. It didn't tip over, but somehow water slopped out over my hand. Albert always does — did — the heavy work like that."

She sniffed and pressed her lips tightly together, almost in tears.

"Maria will dress these burns for you, but I think you should stay in hospital for a day or two."

She nodded.

"I'll go and tell Warren you're here," offered Craig and departed.

The results of the bloodwork on the Mountie were now all back and clearly revealed hepatitis. My impression that he appeared a bit yellow had been correct. I called him and arranged for his admission to hospital and for the rest of the twelve-man detachment to get their gamma globulin shots. These painful injections are given according to the patient's weight; it is usually necessary to put one in each buttock to get the full dose in.

When I went down to start the clinic that afternoon Penelope, the nurse, was weighing a shorter, fatter officer than most of them, while the others looked on.

"I'm not overweight," he pleaded, "I'm under tall."

"Right!" agreed Penelope sarcastically. "You should be seven foot three."

She wrote his weight on a piece of paper and handed it to him.

"Come on in," I called out to him. Extremely reluctantly, he obeyed.

What a performance we had with the whole crew! These fine, upstanding policemen became great blobs of quivering jelly at the very suggestion of needles. Two were so nervous they could hardly walk into the examining room. I decided to wait until Penelope finished the weighing, and get her to help. Despite the moans, even yells, of pain they were soon done and plodded back to their quarters, several with one hand on each buttock.

It was a relief to turn to the next patient, a middle-aged woman with an ingrown toenail that needed removing. She climbed onto the table, took off her socks and never flinched.

After the clinic, I went to the ward to check on Alice and examine her more thoroughly. She was lying quietly in her bed, her bandaged hand in a sling.

"How are you doing?" I asked her. "Do you need anything for pain?"

"No, thank you. It's just sore. The nurses are very kind. Reverend Barnes told Warren I was here and he has been up. It's very awkward for him on those crutches. He always was a bit clumsy. Will it be for long?"

"Another week or so. Then we'll X-ray him again and see. Dr. Paddon thought he might need surgery, but hopes it will heal without it."

"Warren wants me to live with them when I leave the hospital, but I don't know. They only have a little house and their family is so noisy. So was mine, but I was used to it then."

"Don't worry about it for now. Something will work out. Would you like to talk to Dr. Paddon about it? He just left for a meeting in St. John's but will be back in a couple of days."

"Thank you, Doctor."

Next morning, when I had just finished a difficult forceps delivery and was longing for a cup of coffee, Penelope called me.

"I've got a chap here who fell out of a plane," she stated in her clipped British accent. "Can you come and look at him?"

With visions of someone tumbling out of a plane flying overhead, and mindful of the snowplow accident a few weeks earlier, I hurried downstairs. An unhappy young man, obviously in pain, sat there in a wheelchair. Very gingerly he held out his left foot for me to examine.

"What happened?"

"I slipped off the wing while I was doing a routine check," he answered. "It was a bit icy up there. I'm a mechanic at the airport, see."

"How far did you fall?"

"About seven feet, I guess. It was an Otter. Do you think my ankle's broke?"

"I'm afraid so. Let's get an X-ray. Presumably the plane was on the ground at the time?"

"Oh! Yes."

Despite his pain, he enjoyed a good laugh when he realized what I'd half expected. While he was in X-ray I finally got my coffee. His ankle was broken and, by the time I had applied a cast and filled out his Workers' Compensation papers, it was time to start the clinic.

Later that evening Alice died, suddenly but quietly, while sleeping after a light supper. Warren, who had just left after visiting his mother, returned as quickly as his crutches would allow, followed by Craig. Warren looked at me across his mother's bed.

"You know, Doc, this is for the best. Ma would never have settled with us. But how could she have managed at the cabin on her own? Even in summer? Pa did all the heavy work and the trapping. She enjoyed fishing, but she couldn't have handled the boat by herself. No. It's better this way. Bit of a shock though."

"Will you call the rest of the family, or would you like me to?" asked Craig. "You're welcome to come and use my phone again, if that helps."

"Guess I'll be right over to your place, thank you, Reverend.

Three days later, five British airmen drove into the community. They were on their way from England to Omaha on a NATO exercise and had a twenty-four hour stopover at the nearby base. Parking their jeep at the Bay, they pulled their hoods up and set off to explore on foot.

"Everybody must be staying indoors today," remarked one. "We haven't seen a living soul, except for a couple of dogs."

But near the waterfront they came on a long procession. At the head, four men pulled a sled bearing a large coffin covered with bright artificial flowers. Another sled with a smaller coffin followed. The whole community had turned out to escort the couple on their last journey, to the cemetery.

"Who were they?" asked one of the airmen, moved.

"Albert and Alice Anderson," replied a Mountie standing nearby. "Both in their eighties and lived out in the bush several miles from here. No plumbing or electricity. Been there forever; raised their family there and wouldn't come in here, even for the winter. Said it was too crowded and too noisy! The old man had a heart attack and died a few days ago. Then she just died. Real pioneers, they were. The last of their kind, around here anyway."

Two Rescues

Two months later, in early April, I met two more members of the Anderson family. Arriving at the hospital early one morning, I was surprised to see Ralph, the pilot, ready to leave. It was windy and snowing heavily and I had assumed there would be no flying.

"There's a man down at Beaver Creek hurt real bad," he explained in response to my query. "He'll die if I don't get him quick. I won't be long."

"Take one of the nurses, or another man, to help you," I suggested.

He shook his head. "It's illegal to fly in this weather. I don't mind for myself, but I'm not putting anyone else in danger."

He hurried off, quickly disappearing into the blowing snow.

Beaver Creek was a fishing camp about thirty miles from the hospital. Rich tourists came in the summer and fall, but at this time of year I thought the place would be empty. One of the nurses, Stella, filled me in. Two brothers, Milton and Baxter Anderson, were co-owners of the camp, she said, and lived there all winter. Their stove had gone our during the night. The cold awoke Milton, who tried to relight the fire by pouring on a little kerosene. The fire roared to life and in seconds, the whole cabin was ablaze.

Milton got out easily but Baxter, caught in his bunk, was severely burned as he escaped through a window.

"Let's go over to Ralph's and talk to Milton," suggested Stella. "Jeannine will be there, getting him some breakfast, I expect."

As we trudged across to Ralph's house nearby, the strong wind blew the wet snow onto our faces, where it rapidly melted. We stopped in the back porch to try and beat the clinging snow off our parkas before going indoors. Jeannine, Ralph's pregnant wife, welcomed us cheerfully.

"Come in, come in. What a morning! I hate these spring storms. Such a lot of snow they bring! Milton's in the living room by the fire, trying to get warm."

"How are you Jeannine?" I asked. "I guess I may as well cancel today's prenatal clinic?"

"I certainly won't be there. I'm fine, but I'll be glad when I can put this kid down sometimes."

"Won't be long now," said Stella, as we went into the living room where Milton, wrapped in a colourful quilt, sat in an armchair drinking a mug of hot tea. He nodded as I introduced myself.

"Baxter's going to die, you know. He's burned real bad. It's Ralph I'm worrying about. It's not fit to be out."

"Don't be worrying about Ralph," I told him. "What happened?"

"The stove went out in the night. It didn't want to get going again, so I used a drop of kerosene. How many times have I done that? But this time, a big flash came right through the opening in the top of the stove. I jumped out of the way, but it caught something and the whole cabin was on fire. It happened so fast! I yelled to Baxter, but couldn't get to him.

"So I opened the door and ran around the cabin. I bashed in the window by Baxter's bunk and hauled him through it. It wasn't easy and his legs got burned real bad. I could smell his flesh burning!"

Milton shuddered and sat silent for a minute or two.

"We had nothing on but our long underwear. I helped him to the next cabin, got him in a bunk and made him as snug as I could. Then I wrapped myself in a blanket and went outside. It wasn't windy then, so the fire burnt down without catching the trees or the skidoo. With the shovel from the other cabin I threw snow onto the hot spots. Then I came in here to get help."

"The snow's so soft this time of year it was real slow going on the skidoo. Once I was out of the woods the wind got up and I could hardly pick out the trail. Well, I'm here now and that young man, with a wife and a baby coming, is out there. I don't know."

He sighed and shook his head.

"Are you hurt?" I asked him. "Did you get burned at all?"

"Not much," he replied, showing me his hands and wrists, both with minor burns and slight cuts. "My knee is sore though."

When I tried to roll up his longjohns to examine it, he winced and turned grey. I cut away the underwear with a pair of Jeannine's scissors. His leg was swollen and severely bruised just below the knee. It was obviously fractured.

"When did you do this?"

He thought for a moment. "Must has been when I fell down when I first got out the cabin. But I never noticed it till now."

Two male attendants lugged him to the hospital by sled, where an X-ray confirmed my suspicions. Milton must have helped his brother to the other cabin and driven the skidoo with a fractured tibia! I could hardly believe it. As I was about to start applying a cast, Stella ran in to tell me that Ralph was back with Baxter.

Several minutes later, three figures loomed through the snow, two pulling the sled with Baxter on it and Ralph bringing up the rear. Baxter was badly burned, especially his feet. His toenails were burnt off and the soles were a mess. His head and shoulders had escaped the flames, but the rest of him was covered with burns of varying depth. He was alert and calm.

"I never thought even Ralph would make it," he said. "When I saw him come in I figured I was dreaming. He carried me out to the plane like I was a baby. How's Milton?!

I started an intravenous and gave him some morphine, then left the nurses to do the dressings. Ralph was in the staff sitting room sipping coffee.

"You should get a medal, Ralph," I said.

He grinned and shrugged his shoulders. "I went for the lakeshore and followed it down till I got to the creek. Then I followed that up to the camp. I know every tree stump and rock along there. I stayed close to the ground, no more than ten feet up most of the time, or I would have been lost. When I got back here I plunked down on the beach. I was afraid I'd hit a house."

The weather improved the next day and an Armed Forces plane flew Baxter to St. John's. He lived, but he never walked again.

A few months later, in the summer, another life was saved, this time by Rev. Craig Barnes when he flew to a coastal community to conduct a funeral.

That afternoon we received a call on the radio from the Department of Forestry plane. They had a "half-drowned kid" on board, and would be at the dock in a few minutes. Sure enough, ten minutes later the Otter landed on the river, and taxied up to the hospital wharf. A young woman jumped out, and turned to help her very pale, shivering, coughing, and soaking wet little boy. They were followed by Craig. We quickly hustled them up to the hospital, stripped off Bobby's clothes, dried him off and warmed him up.

"He fell out of a dory," explained his mother, "By the time we got him I thought he was gone. But the Reverend brought him back to life!"

"I only did artificial respiration," Craig protested. "It was exhausting! I had just about decided it was too late when he started to breathe again. Do you think he'll be all right?"

"I'm sure he will," I reassured him. Clearly Bobby had inhaled, and swallowed, a lot of water, but physiotherapy and antibiotics would soon put that right.

"It's a miracle," insisted Bobby's mother. "You have got the touch, Reverend."

"Oh, no." Craig was embarrassed. "What I did was first aid. That it worked was God's blessing. You must thank Him, not me."

"I will," she said, fervently, as she left for X-ray with her small son, now looking a bit better.

"All the same, you saved Bobby's life," I told Craig. "He would certainly have been dead by the time he arrived here, even though the plane must have been right there."

"It was. It had come to pick me up. I went down this morning to do a funeral. Well, I'm very happy to have helped save little Bobby's life."

He carried on to his home, while I went to check Bobby's X-ray and arrange his admission.

Plane Crash

The splendid new hospital at St. Anthony was opened in the summer of 1968. Dr. Paddon, with various other important people, flew there for the great occasion, leaving me in charge of our hospital. The very sick asthmatic, admitted the night before, was improving; and the woman in labour was not doing much yet. Everything was quiet, even the clinic.

Early in the afternoon we had a call from the airport. An airliner, with 235 people aboard, would be making an emergency landing shortly. Would we please "stand by." Dorothy, the nurse on duty, informed the few remaining staff, including both ambulance drivers. They were local men, who had worked at the hospital for years, and were familiar with these demands. Bert, alias Santa Claus, took charge.

"Did they tell you what the emergency was?" he asked the receptionist who had taken the call. She shook her head.

"We need to find out," he said, turning to me, "Likely it's a heart attack or a baby borning too soon."

He phoned the airport and spoke to the assistant manager. After listening for a while, he asked what time the plane was expected and hung up.

"Hm, the landing gear stuck half in and half out when they took off from Hamburg; and they haven't been able to shift it. They'll be making a crash landing in about forty minutes."

"They've come all the way from Hamburg like that?!" I exclaimed, "What made them decide to descend on us?"

"They had to use up the fuel to reduce the risk of fire," explained Bert, "And with Goose Bay being a military airport, they can land for free. At St. John's or Halifax they'd have to pay."

Dorothy butted in anxiously.

"But how are we supposed to handle all those people? Where would we put them? There's only Chris and us here, and we can only do so much."

"We'll put them in the waiting room and the corridors," said Bert. "There may not be that many, you know. Some won't be hurt at all, or not much; and some will likely be killed. Don't worry about it. It will be OK."

He turned back to me.

"There's about twenty stretchers, and other emergency stuff in the shed. It don't take a minute to get it. We may as well wait until we know we need it."

He and Tom, the other driver, passed the time reminiscing about earlier emergencies, all involving smaller planes. Just the year before a Cessna had crashed into the trees on the other side of the river, in the middle of winter. Tom, who lived on that side, had gone to the scene with his dog team, and administered first aid to the unconscious pilot. Tom's care saved him from dying of hypothermia until more help could arrive to transport him across the frozen river to the hospital.

The airport called again. The plane was just coming in. Would we proceed with "all available personnel and ambulances" right away. Our one ambulance, with Dorothy and the two drivers, set off. An hour later Bert phoned. The plane had landed and was badly damaged, but there had been no fire. Everyone got out under their own steam, and nobody appeared to be seriously hurt. Whew!

In the end we had four casualties, all German — one with a fractured collarbone, one with cuts to her face, sustained when her glasses broke, one who injured his knee stumbling on the steps as he got out of the plane, and one pregnant woman who was fine.

They all spoke good English, and were soon dealt with. An hour later Tom drove them back to the airport, to join the 231 who were not hurt, to wait for another plane.

As the nurses started wheeling the extra-supply carts back to their cupboard, Dorothy said, "What a relief! That could have been a real disaster."

She turned to me. "You know, Chris, there were not enough staff left here to cope with a big crowd of people. Plane crashes are rare, but it could have been, say, an accident with a school bus, and a lot of local kids needing urgent attention. Or something like that."

"That's true," I agreed. "We were lucky today. I'll talk to Dr. Paddon when he returns and see what he says."

"By the time I had checked the patient with asthma and seen a few patients waiting in the clinic, it was supper time. Shortly afterwards, the woman in labour delivered her baby. We were back to our regular routine.

The Base

The nearby military base was large, with contingents of Brits, Canadians, and, as predicted by the Immigration Officer at Gander, lots of Americans. The British guys came over regularly for cold weather survival training and low level flying exercises. We got to know several of the crews quite well. Before leaving England they would pick up a crate of fresh milk and transport it in the freezing bomb bay of their plane. By the time it reached the hospital it had thawed out, and was seized eagerly by those having difficulty adjusting to "Carnation" and powdered milk. The cheese they brought made a welcome change from the plastic stuff issued by the hospital, too.

Most Saturday evenings one or other of the officers' clubs would be having a party, or showing a movie, and those of us not on duty would troop off to enjoy ourselves. One evening five — two teachers, a nurse, a secretary and I — went with a British crew to the US Officers' Club. The nurse, Dorothy, was Inuit and had grown up in one of the coastal communities. As the British captain signed us in, the doorman pointed at Dorothy.

"She can't come in here. She's coloured!" he declared, loudly.

We were all dumbstruck.

"But she's with us," objected the captain, astonished.

"She's coloured and she's not coming in here!" the American shouted, viciously stabbing with his finger for emphasis.

I was livid.

"Look here!" I almost spat at him, "Out of all the people here, including you, she has the greatest right to be here! She's a native Labradorian!"

The American just stood there smiling complacently. Suddenly, the British captain scratched out our names in the book and marched out, followed by the rest of us.

"Sorry about that," he said. "I thought I was going to hit him, and rearrange that fat face of his."

We were all angry and shaken, except Dorothy, who merely remarked, "I've heard of that happening to my people before."

We went over to the British Officers' Mess, where the men bought us all drinks. Still shocked we sat around a table talking quietly. The Commanding Officer entered, bought himself a drink and joined us.

"You all look very serious," he said. "What's wrong?"

"We just had a nasty experience on the American side," replied the British captain, and told him about it. The CO was astounded, particularly when he heard from Dorothy that it was not an isolated incident. He promised to speak to the US Commanding Officer about it, but I heard no more.

The Wolf

From time to time I did the clinics in the coastal communities. Ralph, the pilot, took off at first light, with me beside him and the homegoing patients on the bench seat behind us. The plane took off on skis from the airstrip in winter, or on pontoons from the river in summer. From my grandstand view in the front of the plane the country looked empty and desolate, especially when smothered by a great eiderdown of snow, on and on for miles with few apparent landmarks. Always, on our arrival, a handful of men would be waiting to ask Ralph if he had seen any caribou, and where.

Once, at an Inuit community over two hours' flight from Goose Bay, we were surprised to be met by four armed men, including the local Mountie and the nursing station janitor. Constable Powell peremptorily ordered me onto the back of an idling skidoo. Too startled to argue (for once) I obeyed. Usually, I walked up to the nursing stations, glad to stretch my legs after the long cramped flight. On the two minute ride I hardly had time to notice that the place was deserted.

At the nursing station Sylvia, the nurse, was watching for me. She beckoned me urgently inside, and the skidoo took off back to the wharf. Grey haired, stocky, and very short, Sylvia barely came up to my shoulder. Looking up at me anxiously, she said, "There's a wolf roaming about. It must be sick or starving; they never come near humans otherwise. The men will have to shoot it. It's no good chasing it away; it'll only come back. So, we are all staying indoors. Come, coffee's on."

When the skidoo returned with Ralph, Sylvia sent the driver to pick up the first patient.

"It will be a bit slow," she told me, "But it's the only way."

As we finished our coffee a loud bang close by shattered the quiet. We rushed to the window, but there was only the usual vista, across the bay to the hills beyond. Then two men appeared, pulling a komatik and escorted by Constable Powell. A dozen other men tagged along. At the nursing station the group came to a halt and gathered round the komatik.

"They'll be wanting you to look at it, and see what's wrong with it," said Sylvia, her brown eyes twinkling up at me as we, and Ralph, pulled our boots on to go outside.

"But I'm not a vet," I protested. "I've never seen a wolf in my life."

"Don't worry. Young Powell will send it to St.John's, to check for rabies, anyway. I wouldn't touch it, if I were you, though, in case it has fleas."

It was a beautiful animal, though very thin. I announced to the small assembly of hopeful looking men that I had never seen a wolf before, and thanked them for showing it to me. They seemed puzzled for a moment, then smiled broadly.

"You take it back and show Dr. Paddon?" suggested one of them.

"Dr. Paddon's away till next week," I replied.

"Can't you tell if it's sick? He would know," piped up another.

"You think I'm as clever as Dr. Paddon? Go on! I just said I never saw a wolf before. Besides, I don't think it's sick; I think it's dead."

They all laughed, then plodded on to the RCMP office. After the clinic I returned home with Ralph, a maternity patient, a man for a TB check, and a sack containing the wolf en route to St. John's.

Next morning Ralph came to me sheepishly, with a cardboard box containing the blood samples I had taken at the clinic. In the excitement over the wolf he had forgotten them, and they had frozen solid in the plane overnight. Our lab technician confirmed that they were useless, and would have to be taken again.

Airlift

On a later trip to the same community Ralph and I traveled in an Otter, as the Beaver was getting serviced. No clinics had been planned for those two days, but Sylvia had called that morning on the radio. A young Inuit woman, seven months pregnant, had haemorrhaged and arrived at the nursing station in a state of collapse. She had now rallied, but clearly needed hospital care. Within the hour Ralph and I were airborne, complete with two units of blood of the patient's type.

Two hours later Sylvia welcomed us, and took me immediately to the small sideroom to see Emily. Despite her deathly pallor she smiled at me.

"She hasn't had any more bleeding," reported Sylvia, who already had an intravenous up, "I've given her two units of Dextran and, yes, I did take the sample for crossmatch first. Her blood pressure has picked up well, but isn't back to normal yet. She's had a few mild contractions, too."

Quickly, I checked Emily. Like Sylvia, I did not do an internal examination for fear of provoking more bleeding.

"Has the baby moved since the bleeding started?" I asked Emily.

She shook her head, her eyes filling with tears.

"Baby dead," she whispered.

"That's what usually happens when you have bad bleeding like this," I told her, as gently as I could.

There were no facilities to crossmatch the blood I had brought, but it was the right type and she obviously needed it badly. I decided to give one unit right away, and have the second run in on the journey. Sylvia and I set it up, then went to her living quarters for lunch.

"It's corned beef hash again, I'm afraid," apologized Sylvia, "Is that what we gave you last time you came?"

"No, we had partridge and it was very good."

"Guess you're getting fed up with canned stuff," remarked Ralph, who was waiting there for us.

"Are we ever!" Sylvia said. "Last so-called summer, as you know, Ralph, the ice never went out of this harbour, and our supply ship couldn't get in. So we had no winter stores this year. The cost of flying goods in is outrageous! It's the fruit and veg I miss more than the meat. We've had a fair bit of caribou and partridge given to us by the community. Now basics like flour are almost gone."

"But it's at least two months before any ships will be able to get in," said Ralph, urgently. "You're going to have to get stuff flown in."

"The Bay promised to send a plane load next week," replied Sylvia. "God knows what it will cost. The people here haven't much cash."

We finished our lunch and returned to Emily, who was looking better. No, she had had no more contractions. While I set up the second unit of blood, Sylvia put together a delivery pack and two small blankets, in case I needed them en route.

Ralph poked his head in the door and beckoned to me. In the hallway stood Constable Powell.

"You going to take Isaac Ford with you?" he inquired as he shook hands.

"Oh! I forgot all about him," cried Sylvia, turning from Emily's bedside. "I don't know if you'll have room."

"What's the matter with him?" I queried.

"He's dead," answered the Mountie, "Went missing a couple of months ago in a blizzard. He went out hunting and never came home. We searched for two days, without a sign of him. Now the snow is melting we've found him - only a quarter mile from his house. He must have missed his way, and fallen down and died. It was very cold and we had a lot of snow that night. He'd have been covered over in minutes. I talked to Dr. Paddon on the radio, and he said he'd have to do an autopsy."

"He was almost home!" I cried. "What a shame! Does he have a family? How old was he?"

"He was forty-two," answered Sylvia. "And married, but they had no children. I've talked to his wife, but she's still in a state of shock. She knew, as we all did, that he must be dead by now. I'm thankful his body has been found, and she knows for sure. Nothing was worse than not knowing what happened. Will you speak to her, Doctor?"

"Yes, of course," I said, sadly following her along the corridor to the waiting room."

Isaac's widow sat in dry-eyed silence as I promised to have her husband returned for his funeral as soon as Dr. Paddon authorized it.

"Yes, miss, thank you," she said politely, and slipped from the room.

"The laundress here is her sister," said Sylvia. "She'll keep me in touch with her."

Ralph joined us.

"Good job we came in the Otter," he noted. "And that I took most of the seats out before we left."

He turned to me.

"You want to sit in that back seat I left, and have Emily on the stretcher alongside you? Then we could put Isaac crossways behind me. Let's get Emily and all your gear aboard, and then decide."

I agreed, and went to explain matters to Emily's anxious husband and mother.

An hour later we were off again. Emily lay quietly on the stretcher, the intravenous hitched onto a hook by the window. Sitting beside her feet on the only seat, with my box of "gear" in front of me, I could see Isaac Ford's wrapped and secured body lying across the plane immediately behind Ralph. Fortunately, Emily was facing towards me. Before we left I had given her a light sedative and, as I hoped, she dozed off.

Suddenly she awoke, and made frantic signals to me. I undid my seat belt, got down on the floor and pulled back her blankets. She bent up her knees, and there were two tiny feet sticking out. There was no time to unpack Sylvia's kit. She had another contraction, and out came the tiny, premature baby, placenta and all. As I expected, the baby was dead. Due to the noise of the plane we couldn't talk; so I just shook my head to her. She nodded and wept a little.

Then I unpacked the kit, and put the delivery equipment aside. The plastic bag intended for the placenta was more than adequate for the baby as well. As I sealed the top I happened to glance up. Ralph was turned in his seat staring at us wide-eyed! I eased a towel under Emily's bottom, added a maternity pad, and covered her up again before she got too cold. Luckily there was very little bleeding. I struggled to my feet and leant over to Ralph, now attending to flying the plane.

"She OK?" he mouthed, as he passed me the radio mike.

I nodded and "raised" the hospital, reported that she had delivered a stillborn baby, and was stable, and that we had a body for autopsy on board.

Another two hours, and Emily was tucked up in bed receiving a third unit of blood; Isaac was in the morgue, along with Emily's baby and placenta; and I was drinking a desperately needed cup of tea, and telling Dr. Paddon about my day.

"There's nothing we could have done to save the baby," he commented thoughtfully. "It probably died at the time of the haemorrhage, which cut off its oxygen supply. It's too bad about Isaac Ford, but these things happen. You've been here long enough to know that, and not to get too upset by these tragedies."

I nodded. Perhaps tomorrow would be a more cheerful day.

Epidemic

That spring a bad flu ran north down the Labrador coast. One non-native community was particularly hard hit. The cook at the nursing station called on the radio to say that everyone was down with it, including the nurse, now lying unconscious on the chesterfield in the sitting room where she had collapsed the night before.

It was late May — "breakup" time — when the ice was not solid enough for a plane to land on. When it melted completely the plane would be fitted with pontoons, but for these two or three weeks, travel to and from the coast was almost impossible. Dr. Paddon appropriated a helicopter assigned to the phone company, and dispatched the public health nurse, another nurse, and me to the community.

My first chopper ride did not endear me to these amazing machines. In the strong wind we lurched from side to side, as the trees waved drunkenly at us from below. Alwyn, the normally garrulous public health nurse, quickly subsided into silence. As we crested the Mealy Mountains she started throwing up and was the picture of abject misery by the time we arrived, forty-five minutes later. Judy and I also had unhappy stomachs, but managed to hang on. All three of us jumped thankfully out into the slush in front of the school where the chopper landed. The pilot was highly amused.

"Sometimes it's worse than that," he said, ghoulishly.

As we unloaded our supplies, a skidoo towing a komatik roared up and drew to a halt right beside us. A young boy, no more than ten years old, leapt off.

"Hello, I'm Skipper," he announced, grinning broadly. "Except for my mom, my Uncle Charlie and me, everybody here is real sick. Even the nurse! How could she get sick? One of you want to ride up behind me? Then I'll come back."

The supplies were loaded onto the komatik, and Judy hopped on behind Skipper. Alwyn and I walked up, glad of the fresh air, in spite of the sloppy ice underfoot.

At the nursing station Skipper's mother Elsie, the cook, welcomed us with cups of tea, then took me to the sitting room. Carole, the station nurse, lay there on the chesterfield, pale as a ghost, her long red hair in disarray on the cushions.

"She hasn't moved since she come in last night. Dare say she's wore out, too. She hasn't stopped these last few days. Everyone's down except me, my brother and Skipper. Must be something in our family, eh? The rest have it though."

Carole stirred feverishly as I undid her shirt to listen to her chest, which was clear. opening her eyes she looked blearily at me.

"Hello, Carole, it's Chris," I said, cheerfully, "Dr. Paddon sent me and Alwyn and Judy to take over. So you relax and drink lots of fluids."

As I was helping her get down a glass of juice Charlie, already introduced in the kitchen, joined us.

"Oh, she's come to. Shall I carry her up to her bed?"

I stood aside and watched with interest. Carole was a big girl, not really tall but much too fat. Charlie was small and skinny like his sister, not much bigger than young Skipper. But he picked Carole up as easily as a baby, and carried her across the hall and up the stairs, followed by Elsie.

By now Judy and Alwyn had checked the inpatients. All of the station's twelve beds were occupied, as were the two cots or camp beds kept for just such a crisis. In the children's room, two of the three cribs had two babies in them. The patients were near-comatose and hardly stirred as I examined them. There was no neck stiffness to suggest meningitis, and only two, both heavy smokers, had noises in their chests.

Elsie looked in.

"We put her to bed in her clothes. That OK? I've got seal meat for your supper. That OK?"

"Is it fresh?" asked Judy, suspiciously.

"It's been in the freezer, miss, it's good," she assured us. "We're out of potatoes, so I'll do spaghetti and canned peas. That OK? About six o'clock? That OK?"

We agreed that would be fine. Alwyn, fully recovered and talking as fast as ever, and I left Judy to care for the inpatients, and set off on our house calls. Charlie and Skipper, each with a skidoo, were ready for us. At Charlie's suggestion he took Alwyn to the houses west of the church, while Skipper took me eastwards. The community was eerily silent. Even the dogs, though unaffected by the virus, didn't bark. Each time Skipper started the skidoo it was like an explosion in the profound quiet.

By supper time we had each visited six homes, where Elsie had said people were really ill. A few needed antibiotics; most, like the inpatients, were feverish and barely conscious, but with no specific signs. After delicious seal meat and spaghetti, followed by blueberry pie, we made plans for the next day. Judy would stay with the inpatients while Alwyn and I visited every house.

Overnight the temperature dropped and the snow and ice froze hard. Getting around was a nightmare, but Skipper and Charlie expertly navigated across the still snow-covered open spaces, as far as possible avoiding the regular paths, which were extremely slippery. In contrast to yesterday's wind the air was still and the sun brilliant, if not very warm.

At each of the homes, mostly small and overcrowded, the scene was the same — everyone lying semiconscious in bed; only the mother, as sick as the others, trying to keep the stove going and get drinks for the family.

Alwyn was startled to find that one of her patients was, in fact, dead. Charlie took the komatik down and brought him to the nursing station, where I examined him. He was an elderly man and his chart indicated a previous bout of TB, and borderline heart failure for the last year. After discussion with Dr. Paddon on the radio, I signed the death certificate: "influenza complicated by heart failure." It was the only death. Even the babies recovered.

Over the next three days people gradually got moving again, wobbly but grateful to be alive. Carole was much better, and tried to help us with the work, until we sent her back to her bed.

On the fifth day the helicopter returned. Leaving Judy behind, but taking Carole with us for a break, we flew home. It was a glorious sunny day. The ride was so smooth we could have been watching it on TV.

American Visitors

All the way from Goose Bay Ralph, the pilot, chatted away, pointing out various landmarks but, because of the noise of the plane, and my inability to lipread, it was all lost on me. Behind me three homegoing patients sat quietly.

Gradually, a speck in the distance developed into a sizable collection of houses, a church, a school, a hospital and a small store. The plane landed on the river and pulled up to the wharf. I scrambled out, watched by the inevitable group of young, very shy, but curious native children. The men ignored me. They had come to ask Ralph if he had seen any caribou and, if so, where. One man left the group and approached me.

"This your luggage, miss?"

He picked up my suitcases, and I followed him to the hospital 200 metres away.

"Here's Dr. Rosenburg," he said, indicating a tall young man coming toward us.

About thirty and very skinny, with straggly, shoulder-length hair and a beard, Dr. Rosenburg was wearing jeans, a tee-shirt, sandals and granny glasses. We shook hands and he shyly told me how pleased he was to see me, and that it was dinnertime.

At dinner I met two of the nurses. Doreen, a stout Englishwoman of about thirty-two, was head nurse and public health nurse. Cathy was younger, a Canadian married to the

Mountie. Joe, the native lab and X-ray technician, was there, too. He told me he'd never seen a woman doctor before.

Leo Rosenburg said he was sure I would be the object of much curiosity. We went up to his apartment in the hospital attic, and he showed me around. I was surprised to see the huge collection of records, mostly guitar, and the even larger collection of books. On closer inspection these proved to be about one-third psychiatry and two-thirds science fiction. Thank goodness I had brought some books with me!

There were four inpatients: one in early labour; one a comatose elderly man who'd had a stroke three days earlier and would clearly die soon; and a small child who had upset boiling water onto himself. The burns to his shoulder and chest were better, but his parents were away fishing, so he would remain with us till their return.

The fourth was a middle-aged man with asthma who had just been admitted. While the aminophylline drip ran into his left hand, his right was busy with a cigarette. The oxygen mask was sitting on top of his head, held in place by a length of elastic.

"He's finally realized if he wants to smoke, he must turn off the oxygen!" said Leo.

The patient grinned sheepishly. "You smoke more than I do."

"I don't have asthma, though," replied Leo, coughing.

By this time, Ralph had taken the three patients who came with me home to their own communities, picked up two more and returned. Leo grabbed his luggage and departed for Goose Bay, en route to Toronto. An American, he had come to Canada to avoid being drafted to Vietnam. In Toronto he would meet his parents for a holiday touring Ontario and Quebec. To set foot in the U.S was to invite arrest. I waved good-bye and got down to work.

There were a couple of babies with diarrhoea to be seen, then the inpatients to check. Later that evening the young woman delivered, and during the night the old man died.

After a week I felt as if I had been there forever, and was well settled into a quiet, fairly slow routine. The patients became used to a woman doctor, and stopped staring at me as if I had descended from outer space.

One beautiful sunny afternoon a child of about eight presented himself at the staff sitting room, where we were all having a cup of tea.

"There's a man down there wants an ambulance."

"What?!" cried Bernice, the nurse on duty. "Who is he?"

"American," said the kid.

Steve, the RCMP officer, came in. "Come on, girls. There's an American having a heart attack in a canoe down there."

Steve, Bernice, and Dan the janitor departed with the stretcher, while I got an intravenous and drugs ready. In a few minutes, they returned with a middle-aged American in jeans, a red-checked shirt and a baseball cap. He was sweaty, breathless, and obviously in pain. While we were undressing and examining him, and putting up the intravenous, I could hear his friend outside. The inevitable crowd of curious onlookers, old and young, had gathered.

"Is this the hospital? My God! When are you going to get the doctor? Huh?"

" Doctor's in there with him now," said Dan, putting away the stretcher.

"She'll look after him. Don't you worry about your friend."

"She! I said a doctor, you dummy! Not a nurse. Get Jack a doctor, right now!"

Steve had been helping us with a patient, but now he went out.

"Constable Macleod, RCMP, sir," he said, in his official voice, "Dr. Rolton's examining Mr. Hawkins right now. She'll speak to you in a minute."

"She!" yelled Mr. Waldo. "You mean the doctor's a woman! I don't think much of that."

"She's been to medical school the same as the men, sir. Perhaps you'd wait in the waiting room, please, sir."

Meantime, the patient had given me a classic history of chest pain, radiating to his left arm, with sweating and breathlessness. His blood pressure was low, and oxygen and morphine improved him considerably.

"Thank you. I feel much better. Don't worry about Bruno. He gets rather excited."

With some trepidation I went and introduced myself to the excited Bruno Waldo. He stared at me in disbelief. I had quickly fallen into Leo's habits, bar the smoking, and wore jeans, tee-shirt and open sandals.

"So you're the doctor! Huh! What about Jack?"

"I think he's had a heart attack."

"Of course he's had a heart attack! I'm not stupid! What does his cardiogram show?"

There were no batteries in the electrocardiogram machine so, obviously, I hadn't done one. I ignored the question and told him Mr. Hawkins was quite a bit better, and would he like to see him for a moment?

"When are you going to get a cardiologist to him? Huh?"

I told him I would call the hospital at Goose Bay and arrange to transfer Mr. Hawkins there, explaining that they had more facilities. Those facilities did not include a cardiologist, but I saw no need to mention that to Mr. Waldo.

"When will that be?"

"Tomorrow, I hope."

"Tomorrow! Aren't you going to do anything tonight? My God! In the United States they'd do something for Jack, I can tell you. And you talk about tomorrow. Tomorrow!"

I told him I would call Goose Bay and escaped before I exploded. What did he expect out in the wilderness? Would small isolated hospitals in the U.S. do any better? I doubted it. By the time I got to the radio at the RCMP I was more or less sane again. The operator at Goose Bay told me there was just enough daylight left to pick up the patient tonight, and he would dispatch Ralph right away. I returned to the hospital feeling positively cheerful.

Mr. Hawkins was stable now, and reasonably comfortable. I told him about the plane coming and he seemed surprised.

"But I'm doing very well here. I feel 100% better. Is it necessary?"

I told him, yes, and he made no further objection. Over the next hour we prepared him for the trip, persuaded Mr. Waldo to bring his canoe up from the wharf, and rounded up two patients who were due to see the dentist.

When Ralph arrived we put the two dentals aboard, to sit in the back, and then loaded on Mr. Hawkins. While Dan, Ralph and Steve were having the usual wrestling match with the stretcher, trying to get it aboard without tipping its occupant into the water, Mr. Waldo noticed the dentals.

"What are they doing here? Get them off. This is our plane."

I told him firmly that they were going too, and that we always used the plane to capacity if we could.

"I'm not having them on my plane I tell you! Get them out of here. Why should they come with us?"

The usually placid Ralph turned on him.

"They're Canadians! This is their plane. Not yours. You shut up or get off!"

Mr. Waldo shut up, and a few minutes later they took off, to the relief of us all.

"He no good," commented a watching child, voicing all our thoughts.

Back at the hospital, I dealt with a young Indian who had been patiently waiting for me to suture his cut foot. Steve reappeared, saying that Dr. Paddon was on the radio from Goose Bay and wanted to speak with me. Over at the RCMP I filled him in on Mr. Hawkins, and gave him some idea of what to expect from Mr. Waldo.

Next day, Dr. Paddon called again to tell me that Jack Hawkins had arrested during the night, and could not be resuscitated. Mr. Waldo was threatening a lawsuit, and demanding that the hospital bring out his canoe and equipment. I was alarmed about the lawsuit, but Dr. Paddon didn't seem too concerned.

"We did all we could. He would have died, anyway, even at a top American hospital like Bruno Waldo keeps telling us about."

A week or so later Doreen asked me to visit Willy, a paraplegic with an indwelling catheter and a fever. His respiration rate was thirty-two, and he had a cough. Like Doreen, I found that his chest was clear, but concluded that he had pneumonia. With some reluctance he agreed to come into hospital, and we promised to send Dan to pick him up.

Doreen and I strolled back to the hospital, reveling in the lovely sunshine while cursing the midges and mosquitoes. A small plane suddenly zoomed in at treetop level and taxied up to the wharf. A middle-aged man in a loud checked shirt, jeans and baseball cap clambered out.

"Oh, no! Not more Americans," muttered Doreen, for we were still talking about Bruno Waldo.

The man spoke to the nearest child.

"Do you have a nurse, or a clinic, honey?"

She pointed at us, so Doreen and I went up and introduced ourselves. We could hear yells and screams coming from the plane, which was rocking on the almost still water.

"There's four of us on a fishing trip, and Bert's been drinking steady ever since we arrived. Couple of days ago our supplies ran out, and he's in a terrible way now. Can you help? We're Americans," he added, superfluously.

Inside the plane an enormous man was thrashing about on the floor, weeping and screaming while two others tried to hold him down. It took the combined efforts of Dan, two other men and the three Americans to get him up to the hospital. He was very tall, and very fat, and hung over both ends of the stretcher. He was in a dreadful state and obviously had DTs. With a pulse of 160, he was pale and sweaty, and terribly agitated. His friends didn't think he had any other health problems, but then they had been previously unaware of his passionate attachment to the bottle. We gave him a large dose of chlordiazepoxide intramuscularly and, when he had quieted down a bit, sneaked up an intravenous.

All this time the other three Americans had been helping us, and trying to calm him. Hank, the one we had spoken to originally, said they would take turns looking after him. They pitched their tents right by the hospital, and were as good as their word. All the nurses had to do was give him medication and change the intravenous fluid bags.

In twenty-four hours we ran out of intramuscular chlor-diazepoxide, but fortunately, he was tractable enough by then to be persuaded to take it orally. On the fourth day he was up and about and eating, though still shaky and easily upset. Later that day they flew away amid good wishes all round.

My last week there was enlivened by a nearby forest fire. It posed no threat to the community, but the comings and goings of the water bombers provided day-long entertain-ment for all of us. They filled up just below us where the river is deeper. The year before on one of the bombers, one door had opened and the other jammed shut. The plane over-turned and the pilot was lucky to get out alive. Each morning most of the population hiked downstream and settled in for the day, hoping for a repeat performance.

On my last evening I was in Leo's apartment packing. There was a tap on the door and Father Leblanc came in. A small Belgian, the priest had been in the community for eight years without a break. They only got holidays every ten years, he told me. He served several communities scattered in the area and was well-liked. Often, patients appeared saying Father had sent them. He was always right, and was very quick to notice an ominous cough, weight loss, or a child "that is not right, Doctor".

Tonight his usually smiling countenance was sad.

"Doctor, we have found Walter."

Walter had gone on a fishing trip ten days earlier and not returned. His canoe had been found a few days ago, so I was not surprised his body had now turned up. With Father I went down to the wharf, where Steve was supervising the removal of the body from a canoe. There were no injuries, so after talking to Dr. Paddon on the radio, I signed the certificate as death due to drowning.

Next day Ralph brought Leo back and my locum was over. Leo had had a haircut, and was smartly dressed in new jeans, new shirt and jacket and new sneakers. He looked well, said he'd had a great trip, and was glad to be back. After dinner Ralph and I plus three patients took off for Goose Bay.

Gaston

The Emergency Department was slow on that cold, wintry evening. Around ten o'clock I was playing Scrabble with the nurse over a cup of tea when the phone rang.

"Uh, oh, wouldn't you know it," Paula said as she got up to answer it. "Hello, Emergency Department — can I help you?"

The voice at the other end was clearly audible to me, several feet from the phone.

"That the 'ospital? Send the ambulance down to the bunkhouse, will ye. There's a fella here real sick."

"What seems to be wrong with him, sir?"

"He's takin' a seizure! Some bad it is, and there's blood coming out of his mouth. His breathing ain't right, either."

"OK, sir, where does the ambulance have to go?"

He gave her directions, while I called the male attendant down from the medical floor, on the other phone.

"Rum fit, most likely, knowing that crowd at the bunk-house," commented Wayne, as he picked up the ambulance keys. He and Paula went off, leaving me alone in the department. I spent a busy twenty minutes getting an intravenous and drugs ready, and checking the crash cart. The evening supervisor, who had been at a delivery, joined me just before the ambulance returned.

The small, pale, dark-haired man on the stretcher was unconscious, but not convulsing. He looked about forty years old, and obviously hadn't shaved for two or three days. The smell of alcohol, vomit and faeces was overwhelming, and his scruffy clothes were filthy. His breathing was deep and noisy, and his lips slightly blue. When we lifted him onto the bed, I put the oxygen mask over his face, and tilted his jaw forward. He soon looked much better.

"He stopped seizuring just before we arrived," said Wayne. "I never saw so many beer bottles in my life. You could hardly get at his bunk. They were everywhere, in the bed and all."

"Don't think we've seen him before," remarked the supervisor, who had worked at the hospital for years. Her husband was one of the first foremen the company had signed on when they opened the mine twenty years earlier. In that northern town near the Quebec border, everything was owned by the mine, including the hospital.

"The other guys said he hadn't been there that long," volunteered Wayne. "His name is Gaston Tremblay and he's from Montreal. They said he was quiet, shy like, and they didn't know much about him."

"Maybe he didn't speak much English," I suggested.

"There was a pile of books by his bed," said Paula, "Westerns mostly, but in English, so I guess that's not the problem."

"No, they said his English was really good," added Wayne, "He wasn't unfriendly, just real quiet. A couple of times last week he went to work drunk. Apparently, he's been drinking nonstop these last two days. Likely, he was fired, I guess."

By this time we had stripped off his filthy clothes and thrown them in the garbage. As Wayne began to wash him off he started seizuring again, a fullblown convulsion. Wishing heartily that I had put up an intravenous while he was quiet, I now had to tackle this moving target. Thanks largely to Paula's expert assistance, I got it the second time, and quickly gave him some diazepam. He settled down, and Wayne went back to his cleanup job while I wrote up the chart.

"Guess we're going to need a special nurse for him," said the supervisor as she left.

I examined the patient in more detail. Aside from his post-convulsion coma, and an appendectomy scar, there was nothing to find. Even his lungs were clear. I wrote up his orders, admitted him to my care and transferred him upstairs.

Next morning he was awake and dubiously contemplating his breakfast tray when I went in. I introduced myself, and asked him if he remembered anything of the previous night.

"No, Doctor, but I must have given you a lot of trouble. Sorry about that."

"No problem, I hope you'll soon be much better. How are you feeling, now?"

"My stomach doesn't feel too good at all. I don't think I want any of this." He indicated the grey glob of porridge and the sad-looking fried egg. I removed them, leaving the apple juice, coffee and toast.

"Try those. Look, I have to go to the OR, so I'll come and talk to you later. Meantime, you can have a bath and get your bloodwork done."

"OK, but I've been through this before. I thought I had it beat. But it's no good."

"Maybe we should do something different this time. We'll see. I'll be back later."

Over the next week we gradually filled in Gaston's life history. Years ago he had had a good job, a wife, children and his own home. He was a respectable and respected citizen. Slowly, the alcohol got a greater and greater stranglehold on him, taking an ever-increasing portion of his paycheck. First he lost his driver's license. Then he was fired from his job. His wife left him, taking the children, and he'd never seen them again. He had to sell his home, and eventually took to the streets.

The Salvation Army came to his rescue, rehabilitated him and restored his self-esteem. For two years he worked with them, helping those caught in the same trap as himself. But he was unable to accept their religion, so he decided to get back into the "real world."

After a series of temporary jobs, he had found a permanent one, a month before, as a labourer at our mine. The lonely life in the bunkhouse and the lack of diversions in a frontier mining town had been his undoing. Fluently bilingual, and obviously educated, he found it difficult to relate to his rough and tough roommates.

Of course, we had no psychiatrist, or even a local branch of the AA. Our own resources were limited to medication and moral support. Gaston was completely destitute, with no money, no clothes, and nowhere to go. At first, he refused to see the local Salvation Army captain.

"They were so good to me, a half-hearted Catholic, and I've let them down."

One day, when the Salvation Army captain was in, Gaston decided to talk to him. As a result, the Salvation Army captain called the Salvation Army in Montreal, who remembered Gaston very well. Of course they would take him back! As soon as they had a vacancy, hopefully in a week or two. In the meantime, we had been pressuring the mining company to take some responsibility for him. After refusing at first to have any more to do with him, they eventually agreed to pay his airfare to Montreal. All this cheered Gaston considerably, but the days were long for him.

When he had been with us for nearly three weeks, we had a call one day from the mine on the Quebec side of the border, thirty miles away along a winding switchback of a road. They had an excellent clinic, with basic lab and X-ray facilities, nurses, a physiotherapist and two doctors. When the miners or their families needed admission they were sent down to us. Most of them didn't speak English, but a few of the hospital staff were more or less bilingual, and there was always a French-speaking patient who would help. Gaston had been a very useful interpreter.

On this particular day, they had a sudden, severe and widespread outbreak of vomiting and diarrhoea. It affected the first sitting in their cafeteria. About a hundred men were ill, said the company official, and would be on their way shortly by bus. We put our disaster plan into effect, with as many staff as we could get together, stretchers, beds etc from all over our small hospital. The medical officer-in-charge told me, as anaesthetist, to just go round sticking up an intravenous in those that needed it, and leave examining the patients in detail to the other three doctors.

Before we were ready, the three buses pulled into the parking lot at the same time. Most of the miners were able to stagger out on their own, to be helped into the hospital by housekeeping staff. Some were in a state of collapse, and had to be carried in. The driver of the first bus walked into the Emergency Department with a pale, sweaty, retching and incontinent miner in his arms. He laid him on the floor in the corridor, the only place available by then.

"It must have been the soup," the driver said, in English. "I had everything else, and I'm not sick at all."

I grabbed an i.v. pole in one hand, and the cart that held needles, bags of fluid etc. in the other, and went to that patient first. Gaston materialized beside me offering assistance. I was puzzled to see he was carrying a hammer and a big box of nails.

"When you run out of poles, where are you going to hang your i.v. bags?" he asked, grinning slightly. I had no time to ponder this or wonder where he got them.

For the next three hours, we went from patient to patient, most of them on the floor, most of them retching, many of them in shock. Gaston was magnificent. He got the intravenous ready, put the tourniquet on, cleaned the site, passed me the needle, tape etc, and talked to each man, in French, reassuringly. In no time, we needed his hammer and nails.

The hospital janitor, seeing this, joined us, and knocked a nail in the wall above each patient's head, for us to hang the i.v.bag on.

Altogether, there were 124 miners in. various stages of shock and dehydration, four of whom had no blood pressure at all and nearly died on us. Finally, we were done and I took Gaston into the OR lounge for a wash and a cup of tea. The medical officer-in-charge was already there with the kettle on. I introduced Gaston and the two men shook hands.

"You must be in this business yourself," said Frank to Gaston, "I saw you giving Chris a hand."

Gaston withdrew into himself, and didn't reply for a minute or two. Then, he said, slowly.

"One time I had my R.N. I was supervisor of the emergency dept of one of the Montreal hospitals. But I blew it with my drinking."

"That's too bad. How long ago was that?"

"Eight years."

"So you don't have a license now, I suppose?"

"No, I'll never get it back now."

I chipped in. "You were fantastic today! It would have taken me more than twice as long without you. Besides, it released a nurse to get on with other work."

Frank said, "You've obviously recovered from this bout. You must find something worthwhile to do, and stay away from the stuff."

Gaston smiled for the first time.

"Yes. I shall go back to my old job in Montreal, and not mind the small income, or the religion. My life isn't over yet."

The Man With The Knife

One afternoon, as I walked into the hospital, I noticed two police cars parked nearby. From the lobby I could see the waiting room beyond. About twenty very tense people sat there, and a Mountie stood in the middle of the floor. Without speaking, he motioned me down the corridor to my right, leading to physiotherapy and X-ray. Glancing to my left, I saw a wild-looking man brandishing a long, thin knife. Untidy dark hair partly obscured his restless, darting eyes.

"I'll kill 'im! I'll kill 'im!" he yelled, cutting at the air with the knife.

Behind him two more Mounties appeared from the front corridor. Hearing them, he whirled round, but they were too quick for him. One grabbed his right wrist hard, making him drop the knife, while the other got him from the back. He struggled a bit, but was soon handcuffed and led away.

"I'll kill 'im!" he shouted once more, as he was taken out the door, "Gimme my knife! It's mine!"

The Mountie in the waiting room picked it up hastily, and dropped it into a plastic bag. He looked around the silent waiting room.

"Did anyone get hurt?" he asked, "Who was here when he arrived?"

"We all were," answered a middle-aged-aged man with his arm in a sling, "He didn't touch anybody, I don't think. He said he was looking for Dr. Walker."

The Mountie nodded and turned to the receptionist, sitting pale and wide-eyed at her desk.

"Could you give me a list of all the adults present? I don't need it now. Later will do."

She nodded, and pointed at the notebook in front of her.

"The ones with ticks by them, they're all here," she whispered, shaking slightly.

Putting the bagged knife down carefully on top of the filing cabinet, he sat down beside her to make a list of the names.

"Will we have to appear in court?" asked the man with the sling.

"I doubt it," replied the Mountie, "I saw enough for myself. But the judge may want a list of witnesses. Before you leave, would you identify yourselves to me, and give me your phone numbers, please. Unless you want to tell me anything, that will be all, thank you."

"OK if I start the clinic?" I asked.

"Sure. Go ahead."

The patients were all surprisingly calm, though one woman was crying, and another still trembling with fright.

"Maybe they'll lock him up now. It's time they did," remarked the man with the sling, as I removed the dressing from his injured hand.

"Has he done this before, then?" I asked, startled.

"No, I don't think so. But he's bad. His wife left him and went back to Newfoundland. Perhaps that set him off."

After the clinic I was in the doctors' lounge, enjoying a welcome cup of tea and checking my lab reports, when Dr. Walker entered.

"Hello, there was a fellow here earlier, looking for you." I greeted him, half-jokingly.

"I heard! Luckily, I was busy in the case room and the Mounties got him first."

He removed his thick glasses and ran a hand through his sparse grey hair. "Maybe they'll put him away for a bit. I hope so. He's dangerous."

"Why was he after you?" I asked, handing him a cup of tea.

"He blames me for the breakup of his marriage. I suppose he's right, really. For months I've been telling his wife to take the kids and go, before she was seriously hurt. She wouldn't charge him. Kidded herself he wouldn't hit her again, I guess. Last month he fractured her jaw, and I had to send her to St. John's. A few days ago I had a note from her, saying she and the kids weren't coming back, and could I send their records to their new G.P."

He drank his tea, thoughtfully, then continued.

"A couple of times in the past, he's gone completely berserk, after getting very thoroughly drunk, and I had to send him to the mental hospital with an RCMP escort. Neither time did he commit any crime, so he couldn't be charged with anything. After a couple of days he settles down and becomes very charming, and sensible, and cons the psychiatrists into letting him go."

He indicated the chart in his hand, and smiled ruefully.

"Would you like to see his discharge letter from six months ago?" he asked, passing it over.

The psychiatrist's letter said, in conclusion: "There is nothing wrong with this pleasant and cooperative man, except marital problems, but his G.P. has delusions that the patient intends to kill him."

"He's tried to kill you before, has he?"

"No, just verbally threatened to. That's the first time I've seen him armed."

"Weren't you afraid?"

"No, but maybe I should have been." He took the chart back, and sat down at the table to write it up.

The RCMP laid several charges against the man, and he was jailed for three years.

Part 2: On To Ontario

By Train and Canoe

$\mathcal{I}$n the early seventies I was doing post-graduate studies in London, Ontario. As part of the course, the residents-in-training worked at remote northern hospitals for a few weeks at a time. To us these trips were a welcome break from the pressures of the teaching hospital milieu; they gave us a chance to be adults again, rather than students. For me, it was a chance to breathe freely again — and not only because my allergies gave me so much trouble further south. As soon as I had completed the mandatory first six months, I put my name down for a stint in the north.

The overnight train journey from Toronto was pleasant enough, but waking to see the sun rise over "Group of Seven" country brought peace to my frazzled soul, and made me feel alive again. My anxiety about giving anaesthetics unsupervised, and dealing with any problems without help, settled somewhat. As I changed trains to proceed yet further north I felt I was on holiday.

The half-empty train plodded along the single track, through mile upon mile of dense spruce trees, which came right up to the line. Poles carrying phone and electricity cables marched beside us.Now and then a small building, belonging to the phone company, would slip by. Although it was early June, there was still snow deep in the woods. Once we stopped, apparently in the middle of nowhere, and two workmen in coveralls and hard hats got down and walked away down a path. As we passed it I could just discern a few houses nestled in the trees about 100 metres away.

A fat, middle-aged woman in a voluminous grey skirt and grubby white blouse came and sat down opposite me. Planting her feet, in their heavy shoes and thick, wrinkly stockings, so wide apart I could see right up to her old-fashioned knickers, she lifted her arms to adjust her grey bun, stretching her shirt to its limit across her large bust. Just as I was concluding she was homosexual, and wondering what on earth she hoped to do on a train, she leaned forward and patted me familiarly on the knee.

Bringing her face close to mine, she whispered, "My dear, are you saved?"

I was so surprised I burst out laughing. She was shocked.

"Oh, my dear, it isn't funny. The Good Lord watches us all every minute. He cares so much, and is so forgiving. He will save you, and all his dear people. Do you want to be saved?"

"No, thanks," I replied, as politely as I could, and turned away to watch the trees and poles passing by.

When I had ignored her for several minutes she sighed sadly, and went in search of more susceptible prey. A young native couple, playing cards across from me, who had been watching with interest, now fell into a passionate embrace. The woman stood there looking at them for a few moments, then moved off down the train. They let go of each other and grinned across to me.

"She's an American lady," the young girl informed me, "She and her friend are missionaries. I don't know where they live, but they often come on this train and try to save us."

"You've found a very good way to put her off," I said.

They laughed and went back to their card game. When I got off the train, I saw the woman and her friend further along the platform. The two were so alike in both features and dress that I abandoned my earlier theory that they were a lesbian couple: I wondered if they were sisters instead.

I had understood that a helicopter would meet the train, to take me the last few miles to the hospital. As there was no sign of it, I went to the station agent's office to ask. From several yards away I could hear a woman's voice, raised arrogantly above the hubbub of arriving and departing passengers and freight. Her accent wasn't British, and I later discovered she was Danish. A harassed looking man was standing behind his desk, his arms spread wide in frustration.

"Mam, I have nothing to do with helicopters or the hospital. There's a pay-phone in the waiting room if you want to call them. Now, excuse me. When the train is in I have a lot of work to do."

The woman, very elegantly dressed and with immaculately waved brown hair, turned and saw me.

"Are YOU going to the hospital?" she asked, aggressive and obviously annoyed.

"I hope so," I answered,"Maybe the helicopter had to go an emergency, and will be along later."

"If they are supposed to meet the train they should be HERE! Do they expect ME to sit and wait for THEM? If their time isn't valuable, mine is. I didn't come all the way from Ottawa to sit around this dirty station, not even MET!"

Clearly she would not be placated, so I said no more. She marched up to the station agent, now busy loading up luggage and checking in passengers. Interrupting his conversation with a couple with two small children boarding the train, she insisted,

"There must be SOME way to get to the hospital. The helicopter obviously isn't coming."

The agent pointed down the street.

"Lady," he said, patiently, "If you walk down there you'll come to the river. Perhaps someone with a boat will take you across."

"How long is the walk?"

"Depends how fast you go."

"And who will take my luggage?"

"Leave it in my office if you don't want to carry it, and I'll put it on the chopper next time it comes, whenever that is."

He turned again to his passengers.

"The service here is APPALLING," she said loudly to his unresponsive back. Then to me, "Come along."

She picked up her large briefcase and small suitcase and strode off down the street. I grabbed my luggage and scampered after her. Though taller and younger than she, I had a hard time keeping up with her. In a few minutes we came to the waterfront. The majestic river flowed smoothly by, mirroring the grey clouds. Small slabs of ice drifted and whirled lazily in the stream. A rocky island with windblown spruce trees blocked the view of the far shore.

Two native men in a canoe drew up to the wharf a few yards from us. She hurried over to them.

"Have you come from the hospital to meet us?" she demanded. Puzzled, they shook their heads.

"Don't you speak English?"

"Oh, yes ma'am, but we're not from the hospital," said the older man.

"Can you take us there?" she asked.

They looked at each other. "OK," agreed the younger.

"Come along!" she beckoned imperiously to me.

The younger man took our luggage and helped us into the boat, while the older man started the engine. I sat on the seat in front of her, hoping to enjoy the scenery, so like Labrador but flatter. As we pulled away from the wharf she suddenly poked me hard in the back.

"Are you a nurse?" she demanded.

"No," I said, and did not enlighten her, still dreaming of a peaceful boat ride. But she would not shut up. To my horror, she started to lecture me in a loud voice.

"These people," she bellowed, indicating our crew, "are so lazy and stupid. They will not DO anything unless you really keep after them. They NEVER learn."

Trying to ignore her, I watched the river as we rounded the island into another channel. Ahead I could just make out a church and two larger buildings — the school and the hospital. As we chugged slowly nearer, houses appeared, and people could be seen walking about. We drew up to the wharf and the older man pointed out the hospital. I turned to my fellow passenger.

"What about paying these men?" I asked. She stared at me in astonishment.

"Don't be ridiculous!" she said, sharply.

The younger man dumped our luggage on the wharf, and helped her out of the canoe. I approached the older man, and gave him a $5 bill.

"I'm not really with her," I explained, so mortified and embarrassed by now that I could barely speak, "Is five dollars OK?"

He nodded, thanked me and leaned a bit closer. "She's been here before. I've seen her. But I never saw you before."

"No," I said, "this is my first visit. I hope to come again."

The men headed back home, leaving us on the wharf. A middle-aged native man, neat in blue jeans and matching jacket, was strolling by.

"Good afternoon," he said, politely. "Are you going to the hospital?"

"Yes, we, are! It's about time somebody met us. We had to take a boat. WHERE was the helicopter?"

I don't know, ma'am. I don't work at the hospital."

She handed him her luggage. He looked a bit surprised but took it, and led the way along the muddy street. At the hospital she headed straight for the nursing office, abandoning me, and her belongings, in the foyer with the Indian.

"I'm not really with her," I apologized again. "As I was coming here too, I tagged along."

"Welcome, and enjoy your stay," he said, smiling as he shook my hand. "I think I've seen her before."

"The boatman thought so, too." I agreed.

As we spoke, the resident I was replacing joined us, and led me off to show me the OR, and my apartment.

"I saw your arrival from the window," he said. "How come the vicar was carrying your luggage?"

"That was the vicar!" I ejaculated, "But it wasn't my things he was carrying; it was that other woman's. She was dreadful, but I don't know who she is."

"The nurses are expecting some inspector from Ottawa, so I imagine that's her. She's been before, and seems to be rather unpopular."

"I'm not surprised!" was all I could say.

For the next two days she was seen (and heard!) all over the hospital, as she criticized everything and humiliated everyone.

One suppertime, I was behind her in the lineup in the cafeteria. She was too busy complaining about the "unattractive presentation" of the food to notice me. Goaded, the food manager burst out.

"They're only going to eat it, ma'am, not pin it on the wall!"

There was a frigid silence. Then a young doctor further back in the line laughed.

"Good for you!" he called out to the manager, who turned an even deeper red, and shifted her feet uncomfortably. Then everyone laughed.

The woman from Ottawa took her tray over to a small table and ate her meal, alone.

"I notice she cleans her plate up," remarked the young doctor, joining me on the other side of the room.

On the third day she returned to Ottawa, to the relief of the whole hospital staff. Even the patients were aware of the relaxation in the tension.

It was a busy two weeks. For the first time in a year an ear, nose and throat surgeon, Dr Jones, was visiting. Patients, many of them children, came from far and wide to get their tonsils out, and other procedures done. In the OR the two male scrub technicians, one Indian and one Inuit, each spoke English as well as their own language. With the children, particularly, they were very helpful, comforting the frightened child in its own language as I inserted the needle; they were also helpful later, when the child awoke in confusion and pain.

One morning Max, the Indian technician, was late. After waiting fifteen minutes, we started without him. The first patient, a ten-year-old girl, spoke English anyway. She was soon asleep and her tonsils out. She was on her way to the recovery room when Max appeared, flustered and out of breath.

"Sorry I'm late. I had to go shoot a bear."

"Shoot a bear! What bear?" exclaimed Dr. Jones, pausing with his hands full of instruments he was sorting to be resterilized.

"My mother called me and said there was a bear trying to get into her house. So I took my gun and went over. It was a big black fellow, and had smashed the kitchen window and was trying to get in. But he was too big. He was so busy he never noticed me, and I got him right behind the eye. Then I had to settle my mother down. She's old and is there by herself. I made her a cup of tea, then called my sister, and she came over. Then I came to work. Sorry I'm late."

"What did you do with the bear?" inquired Dr. Jones.

"Left it on the back step," replied Max. "I'll deal with it after work."

"Won't somebody steal it?"

"A 2000 pound bear! I don't think so. Who would steal it? Native people don't steal — not off each other, anyway," added Max, with a grin. "I'll skin it later. The meat can be cut up and dried, and will feed the dogs all winter. It was a beautiful bear, in good condition, too. I should get a good price from The Bay for the fur."

"How much will they give you for it?" asked Dr. Jones quickly.

"About $200, I'd guess."

"I'll give you $250," offered Dr. Jones.

"Oh. Thank you. But it won't be ready by the time you go. I'll try and get it to you in about a month."

"That's great. If I pay you half now, and half when I receive it, will that be OK?"

Both were highly delighted with their deal and, after a quick coffee, we got on with the operating list.

On the Sunday halfway through my stint, I took myself to the Anglican church. Perched on the high bank of the river, it was small and simple but attractive and had a wonderful view of the surrounding country from the main doorway. The vicar recognised me instantly.

"I hear your travelling companion has returned to Ottawa," he said, smiling as he shook my hand. "Are you from Ottawa also?"

"No, I'm at Western in London," I said. "I only met her at the station. I was so embarrassed by her. I still am!"

"Nothing you can do with people like that," he said easily. "How long are you staying?"

"Till Thursday," I replied. "I'm really enjoying it here. I hope I can come again someday."

Cottage Country Weekend

One summer in the seventies I worked as a GP/anaesthetist in "cottage country" north of Toronto. The resident population was small, and in winter the two clinics were kept barely occupied. In summer time this changed drastically. Cottage owners, living mostly in Toronto, flooded north as soon as school was over, and stayed until Labour Day. Visitors from all over North America descended in large numbers, and it became so busy that each clinic took on two more doctors; one primarily to share the anaesthesia duties with the resident GPs, which is how I came to be there.

The Emergency Department was always staffed by two doctors, one from each clinic. The doctor on first call dealt with all out of area patients, as well as those from their own clinic, and was usually very busy. The other doctor saw only patients from their own clinic.

At 8:00 A.M. on this gloriously sunny Saturday morning in July, I walked into the hospital wondering what the weekend would bring. I was on first call for both anaesthetics and the Emergency Department. On Sunday I would be on for "our" clinic only. Everything was quiet. Nobody at all was in Emergency, except two nurses, one checking the crash cart and the other the drug cupboard. Not expecting that to last, I ambled along to the switchboard for a coffee. I had almost finished it when the call came through.

There was an accident on the highway. "A pile-up!" cried the agitated caller, "Lots of people hurt, send ambulances quick!" My heart sank as the operator tried to calm the caller and get more specific details, particularly about the location. Was it north or south of the town? About how far? Minutes later, all three ambulances screamed and flashed their way out of town, and I went to alert the nurses. They quickly did a dressing change, while I saw a youngster with stomach flu.

One ambulance returned very quickly with an elderly woman and a young man on board. The woman was pale and shaky, and weeping quietly. A few questions revealed that she had only been discharged the day before, from a Toronto hospital after an aortic aneurysm repair, and was on her way home, twenty kilometres further north.

"My husband," she kept saying, "What about my husband?"

As I examined her I promised to try and find out about him. Her belly was tender, especially over the long incision. I ordered blood work and put up an intravenous, and turned my attention to the young man. He was pacing up and down in great distress.

"Oh God! Oh God!" he was shouting, "I killed all those people! Why wasn't I killed? Oh Jesus!"

When I approached him he tried to push me away.

"I'm OK. I'm not hurt. See to all those other people."

"Nobody else is here yet, so I might as well look at you," I said, and led him to a cubicle. He was cradling one wrist in the other hand, and his face was badly cut and his front teeth broken. Making a visible effort to control himself, he told me that the brakes on his big truck failed as he was going downhill round a corner, and he ploughed into a line of traffic coming the other way. I tried to persuade him that things might not be as bad as he supposed, gave him a requisition slip, and sent him to X-ray.

By now the department was full of upset people. Some were looking for relatives; others were just shaken up. A small boy with concussion threw up in the middle of the floor, adding to the confusion. Jim, the doctor on for the other clinic, offered to help and I accepted gratefully, hoping that no other doctors from "my" clinic would appear and accuse him of poaching. Both clinics obsessively guarded their rights to all the business on "their" days, and regularly checked the charts to make sure the other lot were not sabotaging their practice. We summer locums, worked to the bone, often helped each other out and pretended ignorance when caught. Jim, however, was a partner in the other practice. But I realized it would be he, and not I, who would be in trouble.

The ambulance attendants expertly herded everyone but the injured into the waiting room. only six more people were hurt, none seriously, but two people were killed, one of them the husband of the elderly woman I saw first. The other, in the first car to be hit, had to be identified by his dental records.

The young driver who had caused the accident was back with his films. His wrist was badly broken, but his facial bones were OK. I explained that he would need the wrist set, and that we'd tidy up his face while he was asleep, told him not to eat or drink, and went to check the old lady. She was stable, but still asking for her husband. At that point I could only tell her that he wasn't here yet, and try to reassure her.

Then I called our surgeon, Mohammed. Mo was a bit of a prima donna who resented being consulted about patients who did not, in fact, need to go to the OR, and he regarded lesser mortals, notably anaesthetists, as on a par with cockroaches. I told him first about the young driver, then the old lady, and suggested that her anastomosis might be leaking. She was stable, but I was too busy for the endless cross-examination that I knew would follow if I was vague.

By the time he arrived, I was occupied with an unhappy little girl who had been bitten by a rattlesnake. Her foot was very painful, and the swelling went up past her knee. Not having met this emergency before, I asked Jim's advice. He explained about the serum, and how you have to use as much for a child as an adult, as the amount of poison is the same. As she was a visitor to the area, I accepted his offer to take care of her.

To my surprise Mo admitted the old lady for observation without any fuss. Then he asked me to "pass gas" for a caesarian section. After that, he would deal with the truck driver's wrist and facial injuries. I called Paul, my backup, to say that I was going to the OR.

When I returned to Emergency two hours later, the place was blocked. The nurse had called Paul, but he had said they could wait for me. For the next two hours I sutured cuts, ordered tetanus shots, X-rays and blood work, and dealt with earaches, diarrhoea and an asthmatic attack.

Half the crowd in the waiting room were with the last patient, a two-year-old child with week-old burns, for a dressing change. His middle-aged, distinguished-looking father made a point of telling me he was executive director of a major hospital in Chicago. I asked him if he was a doctor, but he said no, he was a lawyer. They were cruising the Great Lakes in his yacht, and the kid had pulled a hot kettle over himself a week earlier, scalding his chest, shoulder and arm. They continued their vacation, stopping off every day or two for a dressing change. The noisy crowd in the waiting room included his children from previous marriages, plus a son-in-law and grandchild, and the little patient, who was the only product of the present match.

One nurse was on a coffee break, of course, so I had to help the remaining one. It was quite a production, with both parents hovering anxiously, wiping the boy's tears and making a big fuss of him. But at last it was done and, to our relief, they all trooped out. They had tried our patience more than a little but, all the same, did not complain about waiting for three hours - I hope because I apologized, and explained the delay, before I knew who they were.

Next, a frantic man with an obviously pregnant wife rushed in in a great state. She was quiet, not at all distressed, almost withdrawn. I spent a very frustrating half-hour trying to figure out the situation. They were from a community 100 kilometres further north, and were on their way home from Toronto, after seeing a gynaecologist, who was admitting her on Monday. She was thirty-six weeks, Rhesus negative, and this was her sixth child. The last child had had several exchange transfusions, but since then the mother had become a Jehovah's Witness. Her husband had not. An hour earlier her waters had broken.

The anxious, voluble little man did his best to give a clear account, but kept interrupting himself to ask if he'd done the right thing, or should he have gone back to Toronto, or on home? She hardly said a word—not that she had much chance. After I had more or less unraveled it all, I examined her. A small foot sticking out confirmed my impression of a breech presentation. She was five centimetres dilated.

I called Paul to pass her over to him, the usual routine, but he was most obstructive, wanting me to send her back to Toronto, or look after her myself. The familiar feeling of being exploited and abused by high-income, fee-for-service physicians, who paid me a salary that amounted to about 25% of my earnings for them, boiled up. It wasn't my fault Paul loathed obstetrics! Trying to keep my temper, I told him I could not take the responsibility. He could send her to Toronto himself, or I could admit her to him. He was furious. Ten minutes later he appeared obviously fuming. Luckily the patient in X-ray had returned, and I got busy applying a cast to a fractured ankle. By the time I had finished the pregnant woman had gone to the caseroom.

Then I got a message to call the jail.

The hospital had been less than popular with the jail since a prisoner had escaped from his hospital room a few weeks earlier. Wearing nothing but a johnny shirt, with an airplane splint on one shoulder, holding his arm out at right angles, he had wriggled through his small second-floor window, dropped to the ground and vanished. The guard at his door didn't hear a thing! Months later, he was picked up in a bar in Sudbury, when the police were searching for someone else.

Today, a prisoner had pain in his side and nausea. Both Paul and I would be busy for a while, so the warden reluctantly agreed to send him over. After examining the young man, I was fairly certain he had appendicitis. His white count confirmed it, so I called Mo, and we took him to the OR.

When I got back from the OR there was another crowd in Emergency, and the ambulance had gone out for someone who had collapsed after a swim. Hoping to get them all sorted out before the ambulance returned, I worked fast, but had only seen three when the swimmer arrived.

A middle-aged man, looking pale and shocky, he denied pain. He insisted that he had fainted and, as he was a physician himself, he would know! Just what I needed! A patient who was a doctor. His blood pressure was low, and he was sweating and taking quick shallow breaths. The monitor showed frequent irregularities, and I turned it so that he could see the screen, thinking that would convince him. But he claimed not to understand "those things," being a pathologist!

I explained to him that he might have had a heart attack, and we should certainly assume that until we knew. He accepted that quite well, and soon had an intravenous up, blood taken, drugs administered, and was looking a good deal better. While the nurse did another EKG, I called Paul, who fancied himself as a cardiologist, and was actually quite good, especially as we didn't have an internist.

He had just delivered the Jehovah's Witness woman, and was arranging transfer of the baby to Toronto. The poor father was in a real bind, as he was not a Jehovah's Witness, but he managed to persuade his wife to agree to the transfer. Paul had to advise them that a judge could order treatment for the baby if they refused. I never heard the outcome.

The pathologist's wife was giving us a hard time, demanding an exact diagnosis, a cardiologist, a private room, a private nurse, and transfer to Hamilton, where they lived. At least twenty times I told her that I thought he'd had a heart attack, and that we would try to get him a private room. But she was extremely persistent. As he had no pain, he couldn't have had a heart attack, so what was wrong with him? she asked.

Paul came down to see her husband and took him over; I got on with other patients, some of whom had been waiting nearly two hours. The nurses were trying to change shifts through all this, and I was getting frazzled, and had not had any supper. One of the outgoing nurses picked me up some chicken and chips, which were delicious and restored me somewhat. I was starving! Paul persuaded the pathologist to stay overnight, with a view to transfer the next day. He was admitted and soon went upstairs.

Suddenly it was quiet! We enjoyed almost an hour's break, which allowed me to recharge my mental batteries.

Then the ambulance went out to pick up a drunk who had stumbled into the path of a car. He was unconscious, covered in blood and not breathing very well. We cleared his mouth and throat, and I put a tube down into his windpipe. His vital signs were normal and his colour improved quickly. Being careful not to move his neck I checked him thoroughly, but was unable to find any injuries, or the source of all the blood. The ambulance men took him off to X-ray and I got on with another patient.

Ten minutes later the ambulance attendant rushed back, and dragged me off to X-ray next door. The patient was sitting up on the X-ray table, triumphantly holding his endotracheal tube at arm's length, and staring around in a dazed way. He coughed up a whole lot of blood and dirt, shook his head vigourously (so much for protecting his neck) and tried to get off the table. The X-rays were done, so we calmed him down, coaxed him back onto the stretcher, and returned to Emergency with him sitting up. The nurse was very much surprised, having last seen him intubated and profoundly comatose. X-rays were negative, except for a broken nose, presumably the source of the blood. He was now alert, talking and very friendly, but efforts to admit him were fruitless.

He had just left, drunk but happy, when a very worried young policeman showed up. "Was that guy who was hit by a car seriously hurt?" he asked, anxiously.

"That was him you just passed in the doorway," I replied. "Concussion and a broken nose. I would have preferred to admit him for observation, but he wouldn't stay."

"That was him! You're kidding! When I first saw him I thought he was dead. Then I realized he was trying to breathe. He sounded like he was drowning. I turned him on his side before I remembered you aren't supposed to move accident victims. I was worried about that after."

"You probably saved his life," I told the policeman. "The car must have struck him right in the face, knocking him out and breaking his nose. Because he was unconscious, the blood from his nose ran back into his windpipe, blocking it. On his side the blood could drain out through his mouth. Anyway, could you check that he's OK later? I wish he had stayed in, for a few hours at least."

"I know where he lives," he volunteered. "I have to get a statement from him. I'll go over there in an hour or two and let you know how he is."

He went back to his duties, leaving both of us much happier.

For the next few hours I was busy with this and that — cuts, sprained ankles, and earaches. By 2:30 A.M. when the place finally emptied, I was exhausted. The chesterfield in the OR lounge was reasonably comfortable, and I soon dozed off.

At 3:15 they called me for an accident. Feeling very groggy, I hurried round to Emergency wondering why I took up medicine, why people had to be out at this hour, why they had to get in an accident and, most of all, why I was the mug on call that particular night. Fortunately, neither patient was badly hurt, and only required sutures and reassurance. I was about to return to the OR, when the police brought in a drunk with a scalp laceration. He was half-anaesthetized already and tolerated the four sutures without local. The police took him to the lockup.

All thought of sleep vanished a few minutes later, when an old man came in with severe chest pain. He was shocky, blue and gasping. I got up an intravenous, put him on oxygen and the monitor and checked the crash cart. Paul appeared just as the patient collapsed completely. In spite of our efforts we could not resuscitate him.

Over a cup of coffee afterwards Paul updated me on his own troubles. He was dealing with a patient we had both seen earlier — the pathologist with the heart attack. He simply would not stabilize, and his wife was really getting on Paul's nerves. She seemed unable to understand that transfer to Hamilton was out of the question until he settled a bit; she still refused to accept the diagnosis, now confirmed.

Paul was planning to call the cardiologist suggested by the patient. If he agreed to the transfer, Paul asked if I would escort the patient while he covered the Emergency Department. Feeling that anything to get out of the hospital for a few hours would be a treat, I agreed willingly. In the almost twenty-four hours I had been on, I had seen sixty-eight patients in Emergency and given three anaesthetics.

It was now Sunday morning, so the other clinic was on first call. I made inpatient rounds, saw a couple of patients in Emergency, and "gassed" another caesarian section. Over the next six hours the pathologist stabilized and, after consultation with Hamilton, the decision was made to transfer him. One of our three ambulances had gone to Toronto with a quadriplegic, a waterskier who had hit a rock doing tricks that morning, and one was out on a call some distance away, leaving only one. So we got a volunteer ambulance from another community sixty kilometres away.

At 4 P.M. we set off with a cranky but fairly stable pathologist and a suitcase of resuscitation equipment. All went smoothly for an hour, though progress was slow due to the very heavy Sunday evening traffic heading back to Toronto. Then the patient complained of nausea. I turned out the drugs, but there was no Gravol, or anything else suitable. We still had a long way to go, so I discussed it with the driver, a very pleasant elementary school principal. He called a nearby hospital on his radio, and they sent the police out with some Gravol, meeting us at an intersection and passing it over. I gave a dose to the patient and we continued on our way.

He went to sleep, giving me a chance to talk to the young attendant, a second-year medical student at the University of Toronto who was home for the summer. For the next hour or so I tried to answer his tough questions, and explain the practical difficulties of the situation. The traffic was unbelievable, and it was 11 P.M. when we got to Hamilton. Our patient had been awake for some time, and was uncomfortable, tired, and fretting about a private room.

Eventually we located the hospital (none of us knew Hamilton except the patient, who was too tired to direct us) and, advised by the nurse in Emergency to go on up, we wheeled into the Coronary Care Unit. The nurses put the patient (still fussing about a private room) into a bed and hooked him up to a monitor, while I talked to the cardiologist, who was there awaiting us. When I told him we found both the patient and his wife rather difficult to deal with, he grinned.

"I bet you did!"

Thankfully, the three of us went back to the ambulance. Tired and starving, we headed for the A and W nearby. It was busy, but the ambulance attracted attention and we were soon served. After eating, and gassing up, we were all set for a peaceful journey home, so I lay down on the stretcher and relaxed. A little while later we were lurching and bumping all over the place. I was jerked awake and tipped off the stretcher. Finally, we got back on smooth road.

"Sorry about that, Doc."

We had been approaching the brow of a hill when two cars came over the top together. Our driver had to pull over sharply, just avoiding a head-on collision. We all settled down again, and I had a nap.

An hour later we stopped for a car on fire at the side of the road. No casualties, so we pressed on. Only minutes later we stopped again.

There was a Volkswagen in the ditch, and bodies all over the place. One was sprawled across the hood, and four others lay not far away. Aside from obvious intoxication they were all perfectly all right, though one became hostile on being roused. We left them there. It was 2:00 A.M. and the roads were deserted.

At the next gas station we stopped for a quick coffee. We were all tired and didn't talk much. A message came over the radio for the ambulance to return to its own community, which meant turning right seven kilometres ahead. The driver/school principal pointed out that they had to take me home. The dispatcher replied that I would have to find another way! The driver laughed when I offered to hitchhike, defibrillator and all. Very generously, he offered to drive me home in his own car. The medical student/attendant said he would come too, to keep the driver awake on his way home.

We proceeded as directed, and had just passed a community when the radio crackled again. A police officer would pick the doctor up at the ambulance station there. So we did a (forbidden) U-turn and entered the small town. The garage was deserted, but the back door was open, so we went in and put on the kettle. Tea was just ready when a sleepy policeman pulled up outside. He had been dragged from his bed, and was very puzzled by the whole business. Over mugs of tea we explained, and I, with my police chauffeur, was soon on my way, arriving at the hospital at 5:30 A.M.

As I handed the equipment over to the supervisor, she said, "I've got eighteen people in Emergency, and they've all been bitten by a boa constrictor. Do you want to deal with it, or shall I call Dr. Bennett?"

For a moment I stared at her. Rattlesnakes, yes, but boa constrictors? She laughed. They were a party up from Toronto for the weekend, she said. One brought a pet boa constrictor that escaped from its cage, and went around and bit everybody! By now I had remembered that boas aren't poisonous; they squeeze their victims to death. She agreed, but said they all wanted tetanus shots!

The weirdest looking group filled the waiting room — long hair, garish make-up, strange clothes. They were high, but happy, presumably on pot, and eagerly showed me their bite marks. Over more coffee at the switchboard I signed the tetanus orders.

Then I went home for breakfast. I was due in the OR at 8:00 A.M.

Part 3: Prairie Interlude.

The Eckharts

My quest to see and experience this vast, wonderful country next took me to the Prairies. I spent several months in a small town set in a large farming area. The hospital had three GPs — Ken Lee from British Columbia, Sethu Patel, born in Kenya but raised in Scotland, and me. The two men both did surgery while I gave the anaesthetics. Patients needing major procedures were transferred to the city two hours drive away, unless the urgency was so great we had to deal with it ourselves.

Our administrator/director of nursing was the stylish, attractive, middle-aged Doris Patoka. Appointed a few months earlier, with glowing references from her previous employers, she had become a serious encumbrance.

On my first day at the hospital she had approached me as I was checking the anaesthetic equipment with a request for Valium, then thought to be harmless and non-addictive. I asked to see her chart. She didn't have one. I told her to get a chart made up, or see me at the clinic. Unexpectedly, she got very angry and told me I was cruel and that she had hoped a woman doctor would be more understanding and respect her privacy more.

Discussing the matter with Ken and Sethu later that day, I found that both had previously granted her request. We all agreed that she be treated the same as other patients — in the clinic with a proper chart and all prescriptions documented.

She mostly ignored me after that, but continued to fawn over the two male doctors, patting their arms as she spoke softly to them.

The following week, Doris, Ken and Sethu attended a meeting in the city while I "minded the store". The two doctors were horrified and embarrassed when Doris got drunk during the lunch hour; she then spent the afternoon session sitting on the floor of the auditorium, singing and burping loudly. On the way home, she threw up in Sethu's car. As she lived alone, they brought her to the hospital, where she slept it off. Next morning, she was back at work, apparently unaware of the stir she had caused.

A month after my arrival, an elderly lady was brought in with a fractured hip. Mrs. Eckhart, aged seventy-six, had slipped on the ice as she hung out the laundry. When told she had a fracture and would have to be transferred to the city for surgery, she became very upset. Who would look after her husband, eighty years old and helpless due to Parkinson's Disease? He was unable to attend to any of his personal needs, even feed himself. I promised her that we would see that he was cared for, then sent her off in the ambulance. Mr. Eckhart was indeed helpless: completely bed and wheelchair bound. Admitted later that day, he accepted the change readily enough, once assured that his wife would be all right.

Next morning, Doris waylaid me as I came out of the OR with an unconscious patient for the recovery room. To her annoyance, we walked right by her and got the patient settled away first. It seemed she would never learn that once patients entered the OR, nothing would take me away from them until they were more or less awake. As I had anticipated, she was unhappy with Mr. Eckhart's admission for "personal care," probably for several weeks. I told her that if she could make suitable arrangements elsewhere, that would be fine with me.

That afternoon, the Eckhart's oldest son called from the city.

"Good afternoon, Doctor, this is Kurt Eckhart. My mother had her surgery this morning and is fine. How is my father?"

"He's settled in very well. We will try and care for him as well as your mother does and keep the routine he's used to as well as we can."

"Thank you so much. How long do you expect Mother to be incapacitated? Can you say?"

"She'll be up and around in a matter of days, but it will be at least six weeks before she can resume full care of your father. He really is very helpless, isn't he, poor man?"

"Yes. I don't know how she does it. Can you keep him at the hospital for that time?"

"I hope so. The administrator feels that his admission to an acute care hospital is inappropriate and is looking into other possibilities, such as a nursing home. If she finds something suitable not too far away, I shall have to agree to his transfer. But that's unlikely at such short notice. If you prefer to make other arrangements yourself, of course, that will be all right with us."

"No indeed. The best thing for Dad is to stay with you, where his friends can visit and read to him. He really enjoys that."

"Someone was in this morning; a neighbour, I believe, who will check the house and feed the cat."

"Great. Thank you again. Will you give him my love and tell him I'll try and get out on the weekend?"

"Sure. Don't worry about him."

On Friday evening, when I was on call and Doris had gone to the city for the weekend, Kurt called again.

"Good evening, Doctor. Mother's surgeon is very pleased with her progress and feels she could be transferred to your care for mobilization. Would that be OK?"

"Probably, but he must call me himself and make the arrangements doctor to doctor, not dump it on you."

"Oh, I guess I'll have to tell him so, will I?"

"Yes. He should know that anyway. Tell him to call me. In the meantime, I'll check with the nursing staff."

Half an hour later the surgeon called and requested the transfer. I asked him if he realized we had no physiotherapist. No problem, he insisted, he would send out the instructions and the nurses could do it all. Knowing how well-liked the Eckharts were in the community, I refrained from telling him the nurses had more than enough to do already, and accepted the transfer.

Before lunch next day, a large station wagon pulled into the hospital parking lot. A tall, heavy, middle-aged man got out and approached Ella, the nurse at the desk.

"Hello, I'm Kurt Eckhart and I have my mother with me. You are expecting her I believe."

"Didn't she come by ambulance?" asked Ella, surprised.

"No. She's so small she can lie flat in the back of my wagon. I can carry her in. Do you have a bed ready for her?"

"Oh, yes, of course. I'll come and give you a hand."

Kurt walked into the hospital with his mother in his arms. As they passed me in the corridor, she smiled and waved, obviously delighted to be back. Kurt laid her on her bed and left her to Ella's care while he visited his father in the next room. Then he came to the desk where I was trying to decipher her very brief, almost unreadable, discharge summary. He introduced himself as he shook hands.

"You know, Doctor, my parents have shared a room for over fifty years to my knowledge. Is there any reason why they can't do so here? Either room looks big enough for both beds. They would be company for each other and Mother wouldn't fret about Dad so much."

"Really, I don't see why not. Ms. Patoka, the administrator, will have a fit on Monday, but we may as well move them in together for the weekend. I'll discuss it with the nurses and see what we can do."

Ella and Janice's eyes opened wide at my suggestion.

"We'd better make sure there's no rules against it," said Ella practically. "But she's already asking for him. We told Kurt to wheel him in, so that they could at least visit."

While they consulted the Policy Manual I went to welcome Mrs. Eckhart. She was lying flat, one hand outstretched to hold her husband's hand, as he sat in his wheelchair beside the bed. A tear rolled slowly down each cheek as he tried to speak to her. She turned her head to include me in her beaming smile.

"Thank you so much for taking me back," she said, as if she had been chucked out for bad behaviour. "They were very kind there, but it was all so strange and big and BUSY! People rushing about all the time. No peace at all."

Ella came into the room bearing the open Policy Manual in her arms.

"It says that 'The inpatient accommodation must be arranged to give privacy to both sexes' but it doesn't say anything at all about putting them in together."

Janice, following her, passed me both patients' charts, which I took to mean the nurses agreed to the move.

"You'd better write on both their order sheets," she said. "Or you-know-who will have our heads on Monday."

As I was doing this, Kurt and the janitor wheeled Mr. Eckhart's bed into the room, placing it alongside his wife's.

"Now I can keep an eye on him. Thank you so much," she said, almost in tears.

"It may be just for the weekend," I warned her. "Ms. Patoka, the boss, will be back Monday and may be able to insist on separating you again."

"That's two days away. I'll worry about it then," she declared, quickly returning to her former brightness. "I knew you would take good care of him, but I couldn't help fretting about him all the same."

On Monday morning I was not surprised to be pounced on by Doris as I went through the hospital door.

"Dr. Rolton!" she bellowed. "How could you order the Eckharts to be put in the same room? Order it! You MUST know that mixing the sexes is not allowed. What were you thinking of?"

"I was thinking of the comfort and well-being of the patients," I replied. "They are very happy with the arrangement, and it's easier for the nurses to care for them together than to keep wheeling him back and forth."

"Oh! Since when did you concern yourself with making things easier for the nurses?" she snapped, rather unfairly I felt. "It's disgraceful! I've already told them to move the old man back into his own room."

Sethu had joined us by now and watched the altercation with raised eyebrows and a slight smile on his usually impassive brown face.

"What's this all aboot?" he asked in his strong Scottish accent. "Something happen on the weekend?"

"Mrs. Eckhart is back for mobilization and I'm letting them share a room. Doris, well, doesn't approve."

"Mixing the sexes is not allowed as you both very well know. I expect your support Dr. Patel. It's disgraceful!"

"What is?" asked Sethu skeptically. "What are they going to get up to? He's totally helpless and she close to it."

"Besides," I added, trying not to laugh. "They promised to behave themselves."

"That's not the point," Doris insisted.

"Then what is the point?" Sethu shrugged his big shoulders and looked down on Doris, puzzled. "What is all this to-do aboot?"

"They have to be moved." Doris was implacable.

"I've written the orders on their charts and I'm not changing them," I said firmly. "If you countermand a doctor's orders I shall report the matter to the Hospital Board."

"So will I," said Sethu. "What a ridiculous fuss!"

She glared at both of us, turned on her heel and marched into her office, slamming the door. Glancing round I saw the nurses and the janitor watching us with bright-eyed interest.

"I have to go to the OR," I told them. "Can you tell the Eckharts they can stay as they are?"

"You bet!"

The couple were with us for nearly two months, happily sharing a room all that time.

Blizzard

Despite living two years in Labrador, I was unprepared for the prairie winter. It thrust out its iron claws at Halloween, and held its grip until Easter. Everything froze hard as temperatures sank to the minus teens and twenties, and remained there. Snowfall was relatively light, but it stayed, unaffected by the brilliant sun which shone day after frigid day. The landscape, flat as the floor, was white from horizon to horizon. Buildings, even large ones such as schools, hospitals and churches, made only tiny pimples on the smooth, empty vista. A passing car, or a barking dog, could be heard for miles.

One weekend we had a blizzard. For several days we followed its progress across the prairies, as it loomed closer. On the Thursday evening news, the weatherman announced confidently that it would hit Friday afternoon around four o'clock. Winds would reach 100-120 kilometres per hour, and between forty and fifty centimetres of snow were expected. On Sunday, around noon, it would clear and the winds drop. Used to the vague forecasts on the east coast and around the Great Lakes, I was amazed when that was exactly what happened.

Between 3:30 and 4:00 P.M., as we hurried to finish the Friday afternoon clinic, the black clouds stole across the previously blue sky. Darkness fell with tropical speed. At 4:15 a few flakes drifted down as I pulled out of the car park. By the time I reached home a mile away, the wind was screaming and the snow whirling down so hard I could barely find my way along the familiar, dead-straight street. My headlights just picked out the reflectors on posts that marked my narrow driveway. I put the car in the garage, plugged it in, and fought my way to the house.

Fortunately, the few patients in our small rural hospital were all on the mend, and crises were unlikely. People scattered around the huge farming area we served, or even in the small town, would be unable to get to the hospital. While looking forward to a quiet weekend on call, I prayed there would be no tragedies — or power outages.

As I prepared my supper, I was startled by a noise out the back. Someone was struggling with the storm door! I ran and opened the inside door. Outside, a small figure was holding onto the storm door with one hand, and hauling my newspaper out of his bag with the other.

"Erik!" I cried. "What are you doing out in this? Come inside!"

I grabbed the storm door, which was threatening to take off into outer space, as Erik stumbled into the house. He was thickly covered with snow, and though well wrapped up, was shivering with cold. I hustled him into the bathroom nearby and made him stand in the tub, while I removed his bag, parka and woolly hat and shook off the snow. Erik then sat on the side of the tub and took his boots off. Getting a better look at him I decided he was OK, though his face and hands were icy.

"I still got one more paper to deliver," he said doggedly, following me through to the kitchen, "It's for the Johannsens just up the street."

"I could keep it for them until the storm is over," I suggested, "Go and phone your mother and tell her where you are. She must be worried to death about you."

Fifteen minutes later, Erik's mightily relieved father turned up on his skidoo.

"Come on!" he growled, rough in his anxiety, "You know better than to be out in this. You're ten years old, and you've lived here all your life! Get your things on and let's get home."

He gave the boy a quick hug, and escorted him to the bathroom to help him dress up again.

"Call and let me know you got home safely," I told Erik's father, as they groped their way down my snow covered back steps to the skidoo, now invisible under a blanket of the pelting snow. They brushed it off, jumped aboard and roared away. They were home in ten minutes.

Later that evening the mayor called. If I needed to go to the hospital during the storm, he said, I was to call this number, and someone would come for me on a skidoo, any time, day or night. "Don't try to drive your car or walk in it," he warned me. The snow was drifting badly, and the windchill was in the minus seventies.

Most of the nurses were local, but we had one new one from India. It occurred to nobody to call Nalini, and tell her not to come, or advise her not to go out at all in the dangerously cold weather. Janice, the nurse on duty over-night, was unable to get home and would continue to care for the patients, but no-one informed Nalini of that.

So, on Saturday morning, while it was still dark, Nalini set out in the raging storm to walk the half mile to the hospital. The wind had blown the road almost clear of snow, except for a hip-high drift across the hospital entrance. By now barely conscious in the desperate cold, Nalini fought her way through the drift, and across the car park. Unable to pull the heavy hospital door open against the wind, she collapsed in the snow.

Mercifully, she was seen by a patient looking out of a window, who alerted Janice. The patient, a big farmer whose diabetes had gone out of control, pushed open the door, and Janice dragged Nalini inside. She was shocked when she recognized her, and soon had her in a bed with the heating blanket on. Nalini revived quickly and, after a hot drink and a short rest, insisted on starting work.

Janice called me, partly to get insulin orders for the diabetic farmer, and asked if it was OK for Nalini to work. I chatted with Nalini for a bit. She sounded fine, if a little chastened. It had simply not crossed her mind that she should stay indoors. She was stunned at the severe cold, having thought she had got used to it over the previous month. I agreed she could work, and let Janice sleep, and told her not to try and go home that night, but to stay at the hospital.

All day Saturday, and through the night, the wind howled, and blew the snow into ever-increasing drifts. The hospital remained quiet, and no new patients came. One member of the kitchen staff, who lived close by, was brought in by skidoo. Otherwise Nalini and Janice cared for the patients on their own. One woman phoned about a small child with a high fever, and another about her sister who had fallen and hurt her wrist. Nalini advised both of them, and told them to come in when the weather allowed.

From time to time I opened my front door and cleared off the top step, in case I had to go out. Otherwise, I spent a very quiet day rereading a favourite book. When the Johannsens, next door but 200 metres away, phoned to see if I was all right, I told them I had their Friday paper.

On Sunday morning the black clouds turned grey, and the wind dropped noticeably. At lunchtime the sun came out very suddenly, flooding vivid light everywhere. The white world was so dazzling I put my sun glasses on to look out the window. In my driveway the wind had blown the snow into a huge cone, taller than the house, but with bare ground around it. The plow trudged down the street, pushing walls of snow into the ditches on each side. Following him were the big scoop and the town truck. The scoop turned into my yard and stopped, and the driver got down. Pulling on my parka, for the temperature was still minus twenty-eight, I went out to the front step. The driver pointed at my mountain.

"Your car in there?" he asked.

"No, my car's in the garage. The wind did that."

"Where do you want me to put it? Down the back?"

"Sure."

I turned back indoors to answer the phone. It was Nalini. Three people had called, needing to be seen. She had told them she'd call me and get back to them. It was now 1:30 P.M. so I said I'd be in from 2:00-4:00 P.M. and for them to come then.

Unable to open the back door, I cleared off the front steps and the path to the now clear driveway. In the intense cold the streets were not slippery at all, and I was soon at the hospital, which was already cleared. Nalini met me at the door, smiling and cheerful, but I stared at her. Her normally dark face was covered in white goo. only her dark eyes and lips were visible.

"My face is really sore," she said, seriously. "Janice put this on it. It's the stuff we use on bedsores. I think I got a bit frostbitten yesterday. It was very stupid of me to come out in that weather. How can the patients trust me, when I'm so ignorant?"

"Don't worry about it," I reassured her, "They know you're an excellent nurse, just not used to the climate here. Anybody here yet, or shall I check the inpatients?"

Over the afternoon six people came in. Five of them had very long Ukrainian surnames, full of zs and ws, which I found impossible to pronounce, let alone spell. As at the clinic, I read the name, sex and date of birth on the chart, and showed it to the most likely patient.

"Is this you?"

"No," the patient would usually reply, "that's him over there."

Again I checked and, satisfied the patient and the chart belonged together, saw to their problems. The last patient, the woman with an injured wrist, was called Smith. She had, she explained, an English grandfather. Her wrist was obviously badly broken, and I admitted her for X-ray and manipulation under anaesthesia the next morning, when we hoped to get back to normal.

Janice cleaned Nalini's face so that I could check her frostbite. It wasn't too bad, fortunately. Two nurses came in, brought by their husbands on skidoos, and took over, enabling Janice to get home to her young family. I took Nalini, who lived alone, home for supper. Aside from the mild frostbite, she was none the worse for her ordeal, though, as I told her, she was lucky not to have paid for her dedication with her life.

Later, as I backed out of the driveway to take her home, I skidded and missed my reflector posts. The back end of my car slid gently into the snow-filled ditch, while the front end barely touched the ground. Neither of us was hurt and we scrambled out quickly. For the first time, it occurred to me that I had not seen a tow truck around town. So I called the hospital, and asked the nurse on duty what I should do.

"Call Thor," she advised promptly. "You know, Sue's husband, who delivers the home heating oil. He'll come."

I thanked her and called Thor. It was now 11:00 P.M. and he had just gone to bed, but he came willingly, rumbling down the dark street in his big delivery truck. Now the back of the car was buried deeply and the front wheels were up in the air. He turned into the driveway, backed up close to the front end, and hitched on a chain. As the nose of the big truck crept into my open garage the car started to move. With a creak and a pop it was out. Thor unhitched it and backed it into the street for me.

"I might as well drop you home, Nalini," he said. "I go right past your place. Hear you were out in the storm yesterday. Are you OK?"

"Oh, yes, thank you. That wasn't very smart of me, was it?"

"You couldn't have known. I guess it doesn't get this cold in India?"

He helped her up into the cab and drove away, waving aside my offer to pay him.

"I'll put it on your oil bill," he said.

He never did.

Next morning I gave two anaesthetics — one to the woman with a broken wrist, and a second to a young girl with appendicitis. She had been ill for over twenty-four hours, but had been unable to get in from an outlying farm. Her mother called the hospital and Janice, back on duty, arranged for a skidoo, pulling a buggy, to fetch her. As soon as we had corrected her dehydration we took her to the OR. Luckily, her appendix had not perforated, and she was soon done.

After the surgery, Ken, Sethu and I were enjoying a quiet coffee with Sue, the OR nurse. Janice joined us, looking concerned.

"You know, Doris still isn't here, and there's no answer at her house. Do you think we should check it out?"

I agreed and the hospital janitor took Sue and me to Doris' nearby house on his skidoo. When we saw the un-touched snow all around the property we feared the worst. After clearing the step we managed to drag the back storm door open. As was usual in that rural area, the back door was not locked, and we were soon into the house. It was empty. She must have gone away for the weekend before the storm broke. In that case, where was she? The roads were cleared and travel was almost back to normal. Back at the hospital we all discussed the matter, and decided to notify the RCMP.

They located her within an hour — at the lockup of the city police! At the height of the storm they had been called to one of the city hotels, where she was creating a disturbance, smashing glasses in the bar, screaming, and trying to attack other patrons. She was now about to appear in court, and would probably be remanded for psychiatric examination. The city police knew her well and so, it turned out, did the mental hospital. For a couple of weeks our hospital jogged along quietly without her. As soon as she was deemed fit to understand, she was fired. Furious, she tried to sue for breach of contract, but the judge refused to hear the case.

The Social Worker

Our social worker, Miss Kunzle, was a strange, middle-aged woman. Obsessive about child abuse and sex education, she seemed to actually enjoy finding possible cases of abuse and to be really disappointed when the accused turned out to be innocent. Also, she would hound unmarried couples living together, visiting them frequently and interrogating them about matters that were none of her business.

She was a member of our local board of doctors, clergy, school principals and others who met occasionally to discuss mutual concerns. At the only meeting I attended, Ken and I were slightly late, and had to take the seats one on each side of Miss Kunzle. She rounded on Ken.

"And WHAT?" she demanded, "are the DOCTORS doing about sex education in the schools?" Her idea of sex education was to tell the kids not to do it.

"Oh," replied Ken, casually, "Chris and I go up there once a week and give a demonstration."

Everyone else roared with laughter, but Miss Kunzle now turned on me.

"This is no joking matter!"

"Actually, I hope the kids can teach me some new tricks," I said, enjoying her reaction. She seethed for the entire meeting.

One day she marched into my office, eyes glittering.

"I have a case of child abuse, doctor," she announced, smiling in her unnerving way, and ushered in two little boys, nine and ten years old, with their puzzled looking father. I knew the family well. These two lads had been born in the same year, the older one in early January, and the younger in late December. Medicare numbers had a family number and your birth year, so these two had the same number. We were always getting their claims back, because the medicare office insisted it was the other one or, when they were both seen the same day, that they were (both) duplicate claims. What did they do about twins, I wondered.

The older boy had a black eye which Miss Kunzle had discovered on a school visit that afternoon. Thrilled, she asked him how he got it.

"My dad poked me in the eye with a hoe," said the kid proudly.

She promptly went into top gear, and brought Dad and the boys to me. The mother was in hospital for surgery, and the younger two children with their grandmother. Anyone less likely to hit a child than this gentle farmer was hard to imagine. Miss Kunzle was livid when I sent her out of the office while I talked to them, and tried to insist she had the right to be there. I just sat there, and she left.

The father explained that he was working in the barn, and didn't realize his son was right behind him. He thought the injury was not serious, so he hadn't brought him along. Had he done wrong? he asked anxiously. I reassured him, and explained that Miss Kunzle believed he had done it deliberately. He was shocked that anyone could think such a thing.

I sent them all out the back way, after checking that she wasn't lurking anywhere, and offered to drive them home after the clinic. In the event, their neighbour was in the grocery store, and gave them a ride.

Then I had Miss Kunzle in again, and informed her that it was an accident, and the injury was minor. When she saw that the family had gone, she was amazed. She really thought she had a case this time, and told me she wouldn't deal with me again. She'd expected a woman to be more alert to child abuse and "such wickedness". With some difficulty, I refrained from telling her that, sometimes, the only "wickedness" was in her mind.

The story ran around the area in no time, and many people commented on the farmer's gentle, kindly ways. One man told me that, if he saw a bird's nest in the field he was ploughing, he'd very carefully pick it up, and carry it to the side of the field, rather than risk hitting it.

The School

One bitterly cold snowy morning, Ken and I were enjoying a well-earned cup of coffee after removing the tonsils from two young children and the gall bladder from a middle-aged woman.

"Hey Chris," said Ken, passing me the cookies, "I think Mrs. Eckhart could go home soon, but I don't see how she could care for the old man yet. Perhaps we could keep him another week to let her get settled and adjusted. Won't that make Doris mad!"

"It seems that threatening to report Doris to the Hospital Board had the desired effect" I said. "I don't see any problem keeping him longer. I'll simply not discharge him."

Sethu joined us.

"How was your meeting last night, Ken?" he asked. "Anything interesting to tell us?"

"Not really. The main topic was the shortage of psychiatrists in the region and delays getting appointments for our patients. It was good to see my friend, Sam, though."

"Who is he?" I inquired.

"Sam is from Jamaica, but has been a GP in Whitcomb for about fifteen years. He is contented enough here, but finds the winters really hard. So do I, come to that. Vancouver is balmy compared to this place."

"Were you born in Vancouver, Ken?" I asked him.

"Oh yes, and so were my parents. Both my grandfathers came from China to build the railway, decided to stay, sent home for wives and settled and raised families. They didn't have it easy. There was a lot of racism in the early days."

"How about now?"

"I can't say it doesn't exist, but it hasn't affected me, I don't believe. Not until last night."

"What happened last night?" asked Sethu, concerned.

Ken refilled his coffee mug and took another cookie.

"I got a real kick in the guts. Hey, do either of you know anything about that school? Victory Academy, it's called. Off the road about fifteen kilometres this side of Whitcomb."

I had never heard of it but Sethu answered. "I know the one you mean. A grim looking place run by American monks. I gather it's pretty spartan and heavy on religion and manual labour."

"Exactly. It used to be a small mental hospital. Can you imagine anyone recovering in those grey buildings in that flat rocky landscape? It looks like the pictures of those Russian gulags."

"What are the Americans doing there?" I asked. "And who goes to the school if it's miles from anywhere?"

"It's a boarding school, run by this American religious order for rich kids — boys — to toughen them up and make men out of them. On the way home last night I had a really troubling experience and I don't know what to do about it."

Ella came in, a patient's chart in her hand. She passed it to me to sign and turned to Sethu.

"Your patient is just about ready, Dr. Patel. Her water's broke and we are moving her into the case room."

Sethu followed her out of the room and I turned to Ken.

"What happened?"

Ken rubbed his cheek — a sure sign he was bothered. "That tedious meeting wasn't over till eleven o'clock, so it must have been eleven-thirty as I was driving past the school. It's about a kilometre from the road, but you can see it for miles in the daylight. At night, it is particularly forbidding. It seems to glare at you across the snow as you drive by. Luckily, I was going slowly. It was windy and the new snow was blowing around, making it difficult to pick out the road sometimes.

"A kilometre or so past the school I saw something small moving ahead of me. As I pulled alongside I realized it was a boy trudging along very slowly. Of course I stopped and opened the passenger door and told him to jump in. He didn't even hear me. I hopped out and round the Jeep, lifted him up by his elbows and shoved him up onto the seat and shut the door. Then I got back in myself, turned the heat up full blast again and switched on the light.

"He was about twelve years old and so cold he wasn't even shivering. Only his breathing showed that he was alive. All he wore were those coarse grey pants and black sweater—that's the school uniform. Sandals on his feet and no mitts or hat!

"As he started to thaw out he took his hands out of his pockets and held them out. He started crying, then howled. I tried to tell him the pain would ease once he got warmed up. After a while he quietened down, but was still weeping. Then he whispered, 'Thank you, mister.' I asked what he was doing, out so late and not properly dressed.

"'I'm running away,' he said. 'I hate that school!'"

"'What was the problem tonight?' I asked him.

"He started crying again. I gave him more tissues. He said, 'I drew a picture to put in with my letter to my mother, and Brother Gordon saw it.' He said it was no good and that drawing pictures was for babies. Then he scrunched it up and put it in the stove.'

"I asked him where his parents were and how he got a bruise I could now see on his forehead.

"'Mom's in Chicago and Dad's in Detroit,' he said. 'They're divorced. The bruise? That's nothing. Brother Stanley hit me with a stick when I got my math wrong. I find math real hard.'

"Satisfied now that he was warmed up and unharmed, I told him I'd have to take him back and he just nodded. So I turned around and headed for the school. What an awful place! It was shut up and no lights showing anywhere. It was hard to believe there were living creatures of any kind there."

"There's a big old-fashioned bell with a rope by the main door. I pulled it three or four times. What a racket! They must have heard it in Whitcomb. I waited and waited. I was about to pull it again when I heard the bolts inside rattling. I helped the boy out of the car as the door was opening.

"A huge man, at least a foot taller than I am, and fat, loomed in the doorway holding an old-fashioned lantern. He wore a black cassock and had long, untidy grey hair and smelt unwashed.

"'What do you want?' he snarled at me. Then he saw the boy. 'Where have you been? Get to bed you snivelling baby!'

"He grabbed him by the shoulder and almost threw him through the inside door. The kid stumbled but didn't fall, then scuttled down the long, dark corridor as fast as he could go. Meanwhile, I had stepped inside and closed the door. At least it was out of the wind. The big monk was not pleased to see me still there. I told him that I had found the boy two kilometres away almost frozen to death and that he needed at least a hot bath and a hot drink.

"'A hot bath and a hot drink!' he exploded. 'Don't you be telling me how to run my school!'

Ken paused, swallowed and put his head in his hands. After a minute he looked up.

"Chris, do you know what he said? He called me a slitty-eyed interfering little chink! Can you imagine? For a moment I thought I was going to throw up, though that may have been the stink of his breath. He needs to see a dentist. Somehow I managed to pull myself together enough to tell him that I and my parents were born in Canada, whereas he wasn't Canadian at all.

"'I'm an American!' he declared in that great harsh voice. If he'd said he was God he couldn't have made it sound grander. Then he flung the door open and shouted, 'Be off with you!'

"It took me nearly two hours to get home because of the blowing snow. Then I couldn't sleep I was so upset — not at his racism — but worrying about that boy and the other kids there.

"How many of them are there?"

"I've no idea. But there's obviously abuse going on, plus the place is freezing and doesn't appear to have even electricity. Surely something should be done about it, but what? It's a private institution and there are no local people working there. In fact, as far as I know, they don't have anything to do with the community at all."

"But they must shop somewhere and go to a post office at least," I pointed out. "Besides, some government department must have issued them a permit to start the school, inspected the building, checked the curriculum. If not, the school can be charged with operating without a licence, housing the boys in unfit quarters, maybe, and child abuse. Everyone physically present in Canada is covered by the Charter of Rights, and bound by Canadian laws. Is it in our practice area?"

"Oh no, it's way over by Whitcomb. It must be in Sam's area though. I'll call him and see what he says."

More cheerful than he'd been all morning, he went to the phone.

At the office two weeks later, Ken, Sethu and I were chatting on our coffee break.

"Hey, do you know what Olav Larsen told me today? You know — the fellow who twisted his knee when he fell off his tractor last week? He asked if I had heard from Dr. Johnson at all. I said, 'No. Why?' and he said, 'Well, when he left he took my wife with him and I just wondered if you'd heard from them.' I was astounded. I never heard about that. Did either of you?"

"Yes. Fiona, my wife, told me," admitted Sethu. "She didn't like either of them and reckoned they deserved each other. What did you tell him, Ken?"

"I said I'd let him know if I had any news of them. He didn't exactly seem concerned about her, I must say."

Sethu and I chuckled. "He must be an odd character," I said. "Or maybe she was — perhaps that's why he didn't mind Dr. Johnson taking her away!"

"Speaking of odd characters, do you remember that episode at Victory Academy?" asked Ken. "Well, Sam called me last night. He's been trying to get the place checked out; he called the Provincial Minister of Education's office. They had never heard of it and sent someone out there. One of the monks chased her away and threatened her with his stick. She was pretty upset, but not hurt, and went back to the city. Her boss called the RCMP and they went there next day. The place was deserted! Just a few schoolbooks and kitchen utensils left. They tried to follow them up, but it seems the whole lot of them returned to the U.S. That was quick work.

"And proof that they were illegal, or at least had something to hide," said Sethu. "Didn't anyone see them go?"

"Weird," I said. "I wonder what will happen to those boys now?"

Ken put his empty mug in the sink. "I guess we'll never know," he said. He was right; we never did.

Reprieve for Blackie

"Chris. It's Nalini. I just dispatched the ambulance to what appears to be a hit and run. Thought I'd let you know."

"Where is the accident?"

"Outside George Popovich's farm. It was the farmer who called and said it was right by his gate."

"That's not far away. I'll be right in."

I got out of bed and dressed quickly. The ambulance pulled into the hospital a few minutes after I got there and two attendants wheeled in a groaning, semiconscious man.

"I think he's more cold than hurt, Doc," said the driver. "Though he does have a bang on his head. George is following us in and will give you more history."

A quick examination revealed normal vital signs and no obvious injuries, except a bruise and ragged gash on his left forehead. He was cold to touch but rapidly recovering consciousness. Leaving him in the care of Nalini and the ambulance attendants, I went to the waiting room to talk to the farmer.

The short, thickset, older man with a fat stomach sat there stroking his dog's head. The big dog jumped up and ran over to me, tail wagging furiously.

Woof, woof, woof!

"Quiet now, Blackie. You'll wake up all the sick people. I was going to give him away, Doctor. He's no use on the farm.

Too friendly. Loves everybody, even the cats out in the barn. Anyhow, I guess tonight he's earned his place.

"What happened?"

"Well, I was in bed asleep and Blackie was outside. He sleeps in the barn. Makes himself a bed in the hay. Anyhow, he woke me up barking under my window. Wouldn't shut up. I thought maybe there was a fox about, casting his greedy eyes on my chickens. So I got up and pulled on my coveralls, picked up my gun and went out. Boy, it's cold! Even for here.

"When I got out there, Blackie was galloping off to the gate. I plodded after him and, as I got there, saw a car with very dim lights parked a little way along the road. It was jacked up. The driver must have been changing the outside back wheel. The tools and spare wheel were lying right there.

"Blackie was barking at me from down in the ditch. Anyhow, I went to look, wishing I'd taken my flashlight. It would have been more use than my gun. I crept down towards Blackie and almost fell over the man. He was moaning a bit, so I knew he was alive and breathing. I touched his head and it was all bloody.

"Anyhow, I went to his car and found a sleeping bag, scrambled back down into the ditch and put it over him. I told Blackie to stay and hurried back to the house and phoned the hospital. Then I put my gun away, picked up my flashlight and went back to him.

"Anyhow, he must have been hit by a passing car, mustn't he? Didn't stop either. That's wicked! Lucky we haven't had a thaw or he'd have drowned in that ditch. It if weren't for Blackie he'd have died, wouldn't he?"

"Yes, indeed. You didn't see anything as you went to bed?"

"No, but that was ten o'clock. I'm up at five so I tuck in early. He can't have been there long. The car battery would have been dead, and so would he. It doesn't take long. Is he hurt much?"

"It doesn't look like it. Hang on while I take a more thorough look at him."

By now the patient, wrapped in the heating blanket, had recovered consciousness but was still a little dazed. At my request, he was able to move all his limbs and wriggle about without pain. His neck movements were full. His only complaint was feeling a bit dizzy and nauseated. I sutured the cut on his forehead and admitted him for observation and X-rays in the morning.

Returning to the waiting room I was again greeted by an exuberant Blackie.

"He should be fine," I told George. "Blackie saved his life."

Blackie wagged his tail and woofed in agreement as he followed his owner out to the truck.

Part 4: Back to Newfoundland.

Outport Locum

An Empty House

In 1980 I moved back to Newfoundland permanently and, for two years, worked in the emergency departments of St. John's hospitals, before starting the locum-motion again.

One March evening in the mid-eighties a Dr. Ali phoned me. Would I do a locum for him for eight weeks, starting mid-April, while he had his gall bladder out? His practice, over 200 miles from St. John's, was centred in a small community and served half a dozen even smaller ones. I asked the usual questions.

Where would I stay? His family were going to St. John's with him, he said, so I could stay at the house. The clinic was in the basement, with a full-time receptionist.

Did he dispense his own drugs? No, he contracted that out to a pharmacist, who also operated out of the basement.

Was he on call all the time? He had an arrangement with another doctor twenty kilometres away for alternate weekends.

What about bloodwork, X-rays and people needing admission to hospital? He took the blood himself, and sent the specimens to the lab, at a cottage hospital, some distance away. The patients went to that same hospital for X-rays. If they needed inpatient care, they went there or into St. John's, depending on the nature of their illness.

Was he expecting a cut towards office expenses? No, he wouldn't take any money, if I would just care for his patients.

We arranged that I would start three weeks hence, driving out on the Monday morning to do a clinic that afternoon. The other doctor would be on call that weekend, and I would take the first weekend after I started.

On the appointed Monday morning I journeyed out from St. John's in intermittent, sometimes heavy, freezing rain. Turning off the TransCanada, I passed through two small communities to my destination. No trouble finding the clinic: a large sign proclaimed "M.Ali, Family Practice and Emergency." I pulled in beside the two cars already there, picked up my briefcase and went in. The pale, middle-aged receptionist was on the phone.

"Yes," she was saying, "Dr. Ali will be gone for a while, but there is a new doctor filling in this afternoon. Two-thirty be OK? See you then, Bye."

I went over and introduced myself.

"Oh. Thank God you've come!" she exclaimed. Her hands trembled, and she seemed upset.

"Why? Is something happening?" I asked, thinking there must be a medical emergency. She shook her curly head.

"Did you think I wouldn't show up?" I persisted, perplexed.

"When I come in here this morning I didn't know what to think," she burst out, "Everything's gone! Oh, I'm Evelyn and this is Don."

The pharmacist had emerged from his cubicle, and now shook hands with me.

"I don't know what to make of it all, either," he said, stroking his luxurious grey mustache with one finger. "Look around."

He indicated the waiting area, empty except for three chairs. Then he showed me the doctor's consulting room with one small table and two chairs. One of the examining rooms was completely empty. The other contained a very old, unsteady-looking examining table and one extremely dirty lamp.

"I poked about in the store room, and found these and set them up," he said, "I think they'll be OK for you. I couldn't see what else to do."

I thanked him and, on a sudden thought, inquired about the upstairs. Neither had been up there — ever. Don and I went up. The stairs came out in the kitchen, which contained the fridge, stove, and one tiny table and chair. Every drawer and cupboard was bare.

In the living room one old armchair sat beside one floor lamp. A single bed stood against the wall in the smallest bedroom. Everywhere else was totally cleaned out. Not a sheet or a towel anywhere. Don stared round in disbelief.

"They've moved out," he said, bewildered. "I thought he was going to St. Clare's to get his gall bladder out."

"That's what he told me, too," I agreed.

Evelyn joined us and gaped around the barren house in amazement.

"Did he give either of you pink slips?" I asked them. Evelyn shook her head. Don said he had a contract with Dr. Ali, and was not actually employed by him.

"How about trying to contact him?" I suggested.

"I don't have a number for him in town," Evelyn replied.

"Someone must have seen the furniture being moved out, surely, " I persevered. "The house is in full view of the store, and the gas station, and about ten other houses. Neither of you saw anything over the weekend?"

But Evelyn lived in the next community, and Don even further away. A grey and white cat suddenly appeared on the kitchen window ledge, meowing loudly. I let it in, and it ran over to the corner by the fridge, clearly wanting food. it looked up at us and meowed again, sadly.

"Oh! What a sin!" cried Evelyn, outraged, "They've left the cat — to starve or freeze! And I thought they were nice people."

Disillusioned and near tears, she sat down quickly on the only chair. I remembered that I had a can of tuna in the box of groceries I'd brought with me, and said so. Don ran down to my car and carried up the box, found the tuna and opened it with his penknife. The only dish was a clean, though chipped ashtray, so he put it in that and the cat wolfed it down.

"They haven't even left you a knife and fork," Don pointed out. "How can you live here? Do you know, they even took the kettle from the clinic?"

I asked about the store just down the street, and was told they sold "everything." Arriving there a few minutes later, I found that to be almost true. Rapidly, I assembled an electric kettle, four mugs, some basic cutlery, and a few dishes. When I introduced myself to the surprised proprietor he readily accepted a cheque.

"I heard he was going for surgery," he said. "But has he gone for good? Without telling us?"

I told him that I didn't know what was happening, but that I, too, understood that he was having surgery. Had he seen them leave? Yes, he had, on Saturday. There was a large, unmarked van there that evening, backed right up to the clinic door so that he couldn't see what was going on, to his chagrin. The van left at 11:00 P.M. and the family followed by car soon afterwards.

"I bin wondering about that ever since," he said, "Are you going to stay, or what?"

I informed him that I'd agreed to come for eight weeks while Dr. Ali had his surgery. During that time I hoped the mystery would be solved. He nodded and packaged up my purchases, and carried them over to the clinic for me. Walking right on up the stairs into the kitchen, he had a quick snoop round. The cat walked over to him and rubbed against his legs.

" She came over to my place yesterday, and I fed her," he

said, picking her up, "I guess you want to move in with me now, do ye? OK, but no chasing the dog. OK?"

I thanked him for everything and he departed, the now purring cat in his arms. Don extricated the new kettle from the boxful of goods.

"Shall I make some tea?" he offered, "They left the teapot, though they took the kettle."

He went on downstairs. I put away my groceries (thank goodness they left the fridge), made a sandwich, and joined Evelyn and Don in the basement.

First Clinic

As we munched our sandwiches I checked the appointment book. There were a dozen names there, mostly women. Evelyn indicated the first two.

"They're just for blood work and to get weighed," she explained, "Though the scales have gone, so how can they get weighed?"

"What's that all about?"

"Well, they are on diets and he has them come in every Monday afternoon for blood work, and to get weighed," she said.

"You'll be doing lots of blood work," volunteered Don, "for all those people taking that stuff for acne."

"What! He's prescribing that drug!"

"I don't know why," said Don. "Their skins look beautiful to me."

He went to his cubicle and brought out a large plastic bottle.

"I go through one of these every week. The patients come on Monday or Tuesday, and he takes their blood, and they get the next week's supply. I've often wondered about it."

I wondered about it, too, and told him to send any unopened bottles back to the supplier, as I never prescribed it. Then I asked Evelyn how they got the blood and urine specimens to the cottage hospital several miles away.

"We keep them in the fridge until somebody's going for an X-ray or an appointment. Sometimes the reports say 'outdated,' and I have to call the patient and get them done again."

"Has he been here long?" I asked her.

"About four years. I thought he liked it here, though she never settled down really. They were real nice, both of them, and the two little girls are darlings, though spoiled rotten."

"He talks like he's British."

"Yes, they're both real dark, but they grew up in England. Her father made a lot of money in oil, she told me. I don't know about his."

A car drew into the parking lot and two young women jumped out, chattering and laughing. Evelyn indicated the first two on the afternoon list.

"That's them," she said. "They always come together."

I went into the consulting room and arranged the contents of my house call bag on one of the shelves. There wasn't room on the minute table, barely big enough for the patient's chart.

"Hi, Evelyn. Did the new doctor come?" cried the taller one. She giggled. "What's he like? Is he young and handsome?"

"It's a lady doctor, Marilyn," replied Evelyn reproachfully. "Hello, Julie. The scales have disappeared, so I guess you won't be able to get weighed today."

"Disappeared? What do you mean?" exclaimed Marilyn, "Hey! The scales aren't the only things to disappear. This place is cleaned out. Has he quit?"

"I don't know," answered Evelyn, helplessly. "He never said." She brought their charts in to me, and sighed. "This is going to be a hard week."

"Don't worry," I assured her. "It will be all over the area

in a couple of days, and you won't have to keep trying to explain."

The two young women crowded into the small room.

"What's going on? Has he left?" asked Marilyn.

I said that he had told me he was going for surgery, and would be away for eight weeks. For that time I would be there.

"Then what?"

I admitted I didn't know, and asked them about the diet they were on. It was just a sensible, low calorie diet and, no, they weren't taking diet pills. They had at first, but then saw something on TV about them, and decided to stop. As there was no scale I couldn't weigh them, and I told them they did not need regular blood work. They were delighted. Did they need to come at all?

"Well," I queried, "When did you last have pap tests?"

They looked at each other. Julie had never had one, and Marilyn not since her postnatal check, over a year ago. I suggested they make appointments sometime in the next eight weeks, preferably when they were mid-cycle. As they departed the quieter one, Julie, turned to me thoughtfully.

"Can a doctor just walk out of his practice, and leave all the people stranded like that?"

"No," I said, as light dawned. "I guess that's why he asked me to come."

"Then you'll get the blame," she said. "That's not fair."

The next three patients were routine - an older woman for a blood pressure check, a man seeing a surgeon in St. John's and needing a referral letter, and a youngster with a bad cough and cold.

Then came four young people, three of them women, taking that "acne pill." They had already been to Don for their refills, but he told them they had to get a new prescription from me. They were the only people in the waiting room. To save saying the same thing four times, I went over to the group. As Don had mentioned, they all had "beautiful skins."

"Aren't you going to give it to us?" asked one of the young

women. "Dr. White won't prescribe it. That's why I come all the way here."

"It's a very powerful drug," I said, "and may cause liver damage and birth defects."

"Oh, we all promised not to get pregnant while we were taking it," said another.

"What about me?" asked the young man, "I'm not going to get pregnant and my pimples were real bad."

"It's a very drastic treatment for what is basically a very trivial condition, unpleasant though it is. I've told Don to send all supplies back to the wholesaler, as I never prescribe it. You can pass that around to anyone you know who takes it. When you've been off it for a week, you should get the blood work done. If that's OK, you need not worry about it."

They all trooped out, promising to return the following week. As I wrote up their charts, I wondered how many times I would have to repeat this, but, in fact, the news soon spread. Evelyn now produced a very welcome cup of tea.

"There's only one more booked," she said, cheerfully, "It's the Salvation Army captain. He gets kidney stone attacks, poor man, and needs some more of his pills."

She handed me his chart. I was startled to see that the patient's name was familiar to me, from my days in the emergency departments in St. John's. He used to come in with an attack and get a shot for the pain, and usually requested a prescription for Demerol pills. Always, he was told to return if the pain was that bad. He claimed he passed the stones but, like the other casualty officers, I was never satisfied he wasn't getting hooked on the Demerol. Don produced his narcotics register. The captain was getting ten pills approximately every three weeks.

"I don't know about him," said Don, stroking that big mustache thoughtfully. "He don't get very much. He can't be hooked on it, can he? That's not even one pill a day."

"He could be hooked on that much," I said. "Or he might be getting them somewhere else as well. I remember him from St. John's, and we wondered about him there. Salvation Army officers, like doctors and pharmacists, are only human."

When the captain arrived, not at all distressed, he recognized me right away, and looked a little crestfallen. I took him into the consulting room, and we chatted a bit about his work and mine, and whether Dr. Ali had quit. Then we turned to his kidney stones.

"You know I don't prescribe Demerol pills," I said. "And you know that you can come any time, day or night, same as in St. John's."

He nodded. As he was going into St. John's the next day, he said, and would be visiting sick people at all the hospitals, would I like him to find out if Dr. Ali was a patient at any of them? I told him I'd appreciate that very much, and he left. I did not see him again during the locum. Maybe he simply had no kidney stone attacks in that time.

Don deposited a bag containing several bottles of pills on my tiny table. Seeing my puzzled frown, he said, "That's for the home. Clarence called and said that's what they needed. You be going there tomorrow?"

"What home?"

"There's a home at South Cove. Dr. Ali goes there every Tuesday morning," said Evelyn, joining us.

"A nursing home?"

"Mm, not really. There's ten men live there. They're not really sick, but I think some of them aren't right in the head."

"It's a personal care home," explained Don, "so it's under Social Services, not the Department of Health. Two of them must be epileptic, one's a diabetic, and three others take medication prescribed by the Mental Hospital."

"That Clarence that runs the place is an ignorant man," said Evelyn. "Always complaining that he shouldn't have to phone in a list of the drugs they need. We should fill them without being reminded. If Don isn't here when he calls, he gets quite rude. But I can't be taking his drug orders."

"All the same," Don interrupted, "He looks after the fellows well, and they all seem content enough."

The phone rang. It was Clarence wanting to know if I'd be going to the home next morning. I took the phone from Evelyn and introduced myself.

"I'm filling in for Dr. Ali for a while. Were you wanting me to come down tomorrow morning?"

"Yes. He always comes Tuesdays, and don't forget the pills! I shouldn't have to do that! The doctor should remember the pills, for God's sake!"

"I have the pills ready here. Are any of the men sick?"

"Not right now. Don't forget the machine to do the blood sugar, and be here by 9:30. Poor Mike can't have his breakfast till that's done."

"Dr. Ali has the blood sugar machine, so I won't be able to do that. Go ahead and give Mike his breakfast, but save the first sample of his water he does in the morning, and I'll test that."

"Don't you have a machine for blood sugar?"

"No, and I can't find Dr. Ali's. He must have it with him. Can you give me directions to your home, please?"

"Just keep on coming to the very last house. If you go any further you'll need a boat, ha, ha. You know where South Cove is, don't you? No? You're a townie, I suppose. Well, you turn down the dirt road just past the school, and it's about ten kilometres."

"Thanks very much. I'll see you about 9:30. Bye"

It was nearly 5:00 P.M. Don locked up his cubicle and gave me the keys, in case I needed anything overnight. Evelyn showed me how to switch the phone over so that I would hear it upstairs, and they departed for their respective homes.

Haemophilia

When I went out to my car for the sleeping bag and pillow that I always carried (in case I was stranded on the road, or needed them for an accident) I realized I had no key to the outside door. Carefully fixing the lock in case it closed behind me, I collected my bedding and returned to the house, locked the door and went upstairs. If I was called out overnight, I would have to leave the door unlocked, and hope for the best. In such a small rural community, it was likely the only house that locked up anyway. I dumped my bedding on the only bed, and went to the kitchen to make a quick supper.

I was exhausted. Was it really only this morning that I had left St. John's, worrying about nothing but the weather? I wondered about this doctor, with his middle-eastern name and posh British accent. What was he up to, clearing out like this, not even leaving a phone number, or any medical equipment behind? Fortunately, I had my own house call bag, and would have to use my own equipment in the clinic as well. Why was he doing weekly blood work on women dieting? For the small fee he could claim from MCP? And why was he prescribing a dangerous drug so freely? Did he have a deal with the drug company? And if so, was it ethical?

Would the patients be difficult about the changes I would inevitably make? Usually I tried not to change things for the patients while their doctor was gone. Here it would be impossible, even if he had been returning, which, obviously, he was not.

The phone rang.

"Hello, this is Bob Simms," said a cheerful voice. "Is that the new doctor? Good. Did Dr. Ali tell you about me?"

No, I replied, but could I help him with something?

"I've got haemophilia, see, and I just banged my knee. So, I need a shot of Factor VIII, and I usually come over to the clinic for it."

"You'd better hang on a minute while I check the fridge."

"I've got the stuff. But sometimes I have a bit of a reaction, and that scares me. So I always come over to the clinic and give it to myself there."

"That's fine. When will you be here?"

"About twenty minutes. Thanks, Doc. See you."

Quickly, I finished my supper and went downstairs and pulled his chart. He was under the care of a specialist in St. John's, but pretty well looked after his disease himself. He had last been to the clinic two weeks earlier. Whatever I thought of Dr. Ali, and some of the things he did, his record keeping was excellent. Everything was documented in clear, neat handwriting. Most unusual!

Bob soon appeared. A burly young man of thirty-two, with thick, shoulder length brown hair and a beard that Santa Claus would have envied, he limped in. Bright blue eyes twinkled at me as he shook hands and said how glad he was somebody would be here while Dr. Ali was gone. We went into the consulting room, and he put his small suitcase down on the table. Then he stopped, and looked around.

"Where's the desk? Hey! The place is cleaned out."

"Yes," I said, "And neither I nor anyone else knows what's going on, yet. He told me he was going for surgery, and would be back in eight weeks."

"That's what he told me," agreed Bob, "You know, I need something bigger than that to set my things up, and give myself my shot."

Picking up the tray of emergency drugs (including adrenalin) that I had put together earlier in the day, I took him into the examining room. I had cleaned off the lamp, and checked the old table which seemed safe enough, for all its decrepit appearance.

"Where did you get that!?" exclaimed Bob. "A museum?"

"Don found it in the storeroom," I explained. "It seems sturdy."

He set out his bottles and made up his solution. Then he sat down and rested his left arm on the table. With his right hand he inserted a needle into a vein, and injected the Factor VIII.

"I leave the needle there for a few minutes, in case you need to give me anything. But I never had a reaction that bad.

Sometimes, I can't get a vein in my left arm. Then Dr. Ali gives it me in my right one. Wish I was ambidextrous."

As he spoke he became very flushed and shook a little. He wiped his brow.

"Now I'm boiling. In a minute I'll start shivering, then I'll be OK."

He was quite right. Within ten minutes he was his cheerful self again; he removed his needle, applied a Band-aid and restored his paraphernalia to the little suitcase. Wondering if there were many people in the practice with this hereditary disease, I asked him if anyone else in his family had it.

"No," he said, "But I'm adopted, see. Did you see about that new test for AIDS? The Red Cross are going to use it to check all blood products now. Sometimes I'm afraid of AIDS, but it's no good bleeding to death worrying about something that will probably never happen, is it? If Dr. Ali has left, and he must have done, will you stay?"

I shook my head, and explained that I did locums all the time, filling in for sick or vacationing doctors all over the province.

"That must be more interesting than seeing the same old faces all the time," he said, thoughtfully. "But isn't it difficult dealing with patients you don't know?"

"Sometimes. Then someone like you comes along and makes my day."

"Thanks! Well, Doc, I guess I'll see you again. Thanks a lot."

"You'll be able to replace your supplies yourself, will you?"

"Oh, yes, I'll call the Red Cross in the morning. Bye now. Thanks again."

He limped back to his truck cheerfully, and I returned upstairs heartened, made a cup of tea and relaxed. There were no more calls that night.

South Cove

Next morning Don arrived first and let himself into the clinic. I went down to return his keys and pointed out that I had no house key, and would have had to leave the house open if I had been called out.

"I'll give you mine, I guess, and you can let me in each morning," he suggested. "That shouldn't be a problem. Evelyn has a key, too. Maybe she could get another cut on the weekend. Here she is."

"Morning," Evelyn greeted us. "I bought some coffee and teabags and milk on my way. That's why I'm a bit late. Did you have any calls last night?"

"Bob Simms came over. I left his chart out so that you can file an MCP claim, please."

"Did he come after six? Yes? That's a different code. You get a bit more, too."

Picking up my house call bag, the pills, and the bundle of charts Evelyn had put out the evening before, I departed for South Cove, turning off just past the school, as directed. The winding dirt road was wet and full of potholes, but the scenery was spectacular. On my right the densely packed spruce trees gave way to towering cliffs. On my left I could see right across the glittering bay to two small communities on the far side. An osprey, with a large fish in its claws, flew by only a few feet away.

Unexpectedly, the cliffs came to an end, revealing green meadows, a small cove and about twenty houses dotted around it. The road ended abruptly at a tiny beach, and I almost drove into the water. Off to the left stood a big, plain two-storey house. Three young men were playing ball on the grass outside, assisted by a large, nondescript dog that ran back and forth as they threw the ball. I backed up and turned into the driveway, pulling up beside a battered old station wagon.

As I got out of the car, the dog rushed up to me, barking

loudly, and rubbed his muddy self against my clean pants. One of the young men came over, stumbling with the typical gait of a cerebral palsy victim. Making noises and shaking his head and pointing at the dog, he was obviously trying to tell me that the dog wouldn't hurt me. The other two ball players joined us. Both were short and stocky and had Down's syndrome, and big smiles. The older of the two peered closely into my face.

"You lady doctor?" he asked.

"Yes," I answered, "Shall we go indoors?"

Taking my hand, he led me up the back steps into the kitchen, where a youngish woman was sweeping up some broken china. A large, bald, middle-aged man, his shirt open to reveal his hairy chest and paunch, entered from the hall. Without removing the cigarette from his mouth, he offered his hand.

"Morning, Doctor, I'm Clarence Butler. Come in, come in."

He noticed my mucky pants and frowned.

"Did you fall down?"

"Dog did it," said the man with Down's, still holding my hand and smiling.

"He was only being friendly," I assured him, hastily. Clarence shooed the men and the dog outdoors, and took me into his small office.

"Did you bring the pills? Good. What do you take in your coffee?"

By the time he returned with two steaming mugs, I had set out my stethoscope and blood pressure apparatus and was checking the urine sample with a "dipstick."

"This must be Mike's," I said. "Just a trace of sugar, which is fine."

"Why did Dr. Ali take his machine with him, if he's gone for surgery? He's not diabetic, as far as I know."

"I don't know," I said. "Tell me about your fellows."

He had two who were awaiting surgery at the Grace

Hospital. Did I have any news about when they would be going in? I checked their charts. Nothing. Would I, Clarence asked, be able to arrange for them to go in at the same time? It would be easier for him, driving them back and forth, and they'd be company for each other. Both were awaiting hernia repair, and would be under the same surgeon. I promised to call the surgeon and see what I could fix up. I suggested I check both men.

"Hm," said Clarence. "They might be shy about taking their pants down in front of a lady. They weren't that keen to show Dr. Ali, either of them."

"He has seen them, though?"

"Oh, yes."

I finished my coffee and saw each of the ten men in the home. All had varying degrees of retardation, and about half had other medical problems, too. They were all clean, happy, and obviously had a good relationship with Clarence, who gently bullied them into taking their shirts off, letting me take their blood pressures and so on. One tiny older man kept trying to kiss me, and had to be physically removed by Clarence.

"Come on, Bernie, let the doctor be. Or I'll beat you black and blue with a baseball bat!"

Bernie laughed and sat down.

"I always tell them that," explained Clarence. "But I don't even have a baseball bat."

"I'm sure you'd never dream of doing such a thing," I said, for this rather odd man was clearly very fond of his charges. "Any more?"

"No, thanks Doc. You'll let me know about Terry and Brian, won't you?"

I agreed and departed. The drive back was rather dreary. All I could see was the grey, choppy water and the cliffs, then the spruce trees. The sky had clouded over, and it was raining lightly, and very gloomy.

The afternoon clinic was busy with the usual blood pressure checks, coughs, colds and backaches. One older, diabetic man needed an abscess in his armpit lanced. Two women came for pap tests and breast exams, having already heard that a woman doctor was in Dr. Ali's place. Both remarked that it was much less stressful with a woman doctor, and that I would be busy. I was.

I called the surgeon in St. John's about the two men at the home in South Cove, explaining the advantages of them both coming in together. He offered to admit them the following Wednesday for surgery on Thursday, and asked would I notify Clarence. I thanked him and called Clarence, who was delighted at the news.

That night the only call was from the Salvation Army captain, just returned from St. John's. Dr. Ali was not a patient at any of the hospitals. He had even checked at the Mental Hospital, as he had visited someone there.

Next morning I called the Newfoundland Medical Association and spoke to the CEO, an old friend. Yes, he had recommended me to Dr. Ali, and lots of other doctors, too. I was a very useful person, he said, one of the most popular in the province, at least among the GPs. I thanked him for his kind words, and asked him what he understood the situation with Dr. Ali to be. Like everyone else, he thought Dr. Ali was getting his gall bladder out, and was amazed when I told him about the empty house and clinic, and the abandoned cat. He promised to investigate.

The week ground on, moderately busy, with only two evening calls, and no night work at all. The weekend changed all that, as I covered Dr.White's practice as well as Dr. Ali's.

Weekend On Call

At 8:00 A.M. Saturday morning, as I was enjoying my second mug of tea, the phone rang. The caller's ninety-year-old mother had fallen and hurt her shoulder. Could he bring her over? A few minutes later they arrived, followed closely by an ambulance. Two cars had collided at a quiet intersection where neither driver had expected to meet any other traffic.

I checked the drivers first. One, an older man, moaned and clutched his head. He seemed dazed, but not seriously hurt. The other driver, a young woman, was supporting her right wrist and weeping.

"It wasn't my fault," she maintained. "I was on the main road, and he jumped out at me."

The ambulance driver nodded confirmation of this. Both patients needed X-rays, so I sent them on to the cottage hospital. I turned to the old lady, still sitting in her son's car.

"I tripped over the back step, and landed against the kitchen table," she raged. "I've lived in that house for sixty years! You'd think I'd know where the back step is by now, wouldn't you? Have I broke my shoulder?"

I thought so, and sent her on to the cottage hospital, too. Then I phoned them to warn them to expect three patients, all with probable broken bones. The young doctor had a quiet South African accent, and was very helpful. How was I getting on there, he asked? Was it true that Dr. Ali had quit, leaving me with no equipment or furniture? The lab really noticed the difference. He'd be happy to see the patients I'd sent. It sounded as if we were both in for a busy weekend, didn't it?

There were no more patients until the middle of the afternoon, when a couple showed up with their German shepherd. They'd found him unconscious by the side of the road, they explained. Did I think he'd been hit by a car? In the back of their station wagon the dog was lying comfortably, as if asleep. There were no apparent injuries, but he didn't stir as I examined him gently. As I knew that the only vet between us and St. John's was away, I told them to take him into town, then phone round the vets until they were able to contact one.

Early on Sunday morning a woman phoned.

"My sister's got an awful pain in her stomach," she stated. "Can I bring her along, please?"

Half an hour later they pulled in, and a very pregnant woman waddled into the clinic. When I asked her if she was a patient of Dr. White's, she shrugged.

"I haven't been to the doctor. I've been feeling grand, see."

Clearly she was in early labour, but examination revealed that dilatation had barely started. I called the ambulance to take her into St. John's. The very young driver strode cheerfully into the waiting room to collect her. She stared at him, her face flushing.

"You!" she gasped.

He gazed back at her, startled but not put out.

"Hi, Cindy. You coming for a ride in my bus?"

"I suppose so. I didn't know you were driving the ambulance."

"I hadn't heard you were back home. Where you been this last year? Toronto?"

She nodded.

"Big place, Toronto," he said, easily. "All sorts of things happen there." He turned to me. "Where are we going? The Grace or St.Clare's?"

"The Grace," I replied. "Good luck, Cindy."

The rest of the day was slow, but by Monday morning I had seen nineteen patients, eight of them "belonging" to Dr. White. Before starting the clinic I called him about them, particularly two older people who needed to be followed up. I also mentioned one elderly man that I had sent to the cottage hospital with chest pain. He had never had angina, and was previously in good health.

"Oh, I know him," said Dr. White, "I haven't seen him for a year or more. He was the sheepshooter."

The what?

"Years ago the sheep in Newfoundland got a dreadful disease. We called it bluebottle fly disease. The bluebottles laid their eggs in the wool, transmitting the bug. It ate through the sheep's skins right into their guts. The government ordered them all to be shot, and appointed Ernest the sheepshooter. About thirty years ago that was, when I was a boy. How are you getting on there? Is it true Ali's quit?"

I told him that it appeared that way, but I didn't know for sure, and hung up.

Bernie.

The week was fairly busy. All eighteen patients on the "acne pill" dutifully came in for their blood work, most of them on Monday afternoon. The last one was going to the cottage hospital to visit her mother, and offered to take the samples with her. I accepted gratefully, and packed them all up carefully, in a box provided by Don.

On Thursday morning Clarence appeared, carrying Bernie, the old man who had tried to kiss me on my first visit to the home, in his arms. He laid him on the examining table.

"This thing safe?" he asked, giving the table a shake. "Hm, seems to be."

He indicated the unconscious, snoring Bernie. "Good thing I DON'T have a baseball bat, I tell you! Not for him, he don't know any better, but for his damn sister!"

"His sister?"

"Yesterday, I drove into St. John's to take Terry and Brian to the Grace. Bernie and two of the other fellows came with us. They love an outing, and they play Mrs. Parsons up when she looks after them. The others are no trouble with her.

"Well, we took Terry and Brian to the Grace, and got them settled in. Then we went to the mall. Bernie slipped away on me. He'd seen his sister, quite by chance, see. She lives in St. John's. Do you know what that silly woman did?"

His voice rose angrily. "She took him to the liquor store, and bought him a bottle of rum! She's got no more brains than he has! He put it in the pocket of that big old coat he wears, and never said. On the way home he got it out, and drank the whole lot down before I realized what he was up to. He was sitting in the back of the car, see. I pulled over and got him out, and walked him up and down, and bent him over and smacked him on the back, and he threw up most of it. Just before we got home he threw up again, all over the back seat of the car. You can still smell it, though I chucked the blanket that got most of it. When he comes to he just holds his head and groans. I guess he's hungover, but I figured I'd better get him checked out."

There was no window in the tiny room, so I opened the door before the fumes of stale alcohol suffocated us all. Bernie was a bit dehydrated. As I tested for neck stiffness, he whimpered and try to push me away. Clarence held his wrists as I examined his abdomen, then let him sit up. He looked around blearily, shook his head, then grabbed it and moaned. He tried to get off the table, so we helped him down. He stood unsteadily, clutching Clarence's arm.

"Walk him over to the chair there in the waiting room, and let him sit down," I instructed Clarence.

Bernie walked quite well, and I was satisfied he hadn't had a stroke or other catastrophe. Then he let me take his blood pressure, which was normal.

"Has he kept any fluids down?" I asked Clarence.

"Just a glass of ginger ale this morning. Should I try to make him drink? I didn't give him his epileptic pills this morning, as I thought he might throw them up."

"How long since he had a seizure?"

"Years. He's only had two all the time he's been with me."

"OK. Hold his pills today and start them again tomorrow. Make him drink as much as you can — ginger ale, juice, water, milk — anything nonalcoholic. And walk him about from time to time. If you're not happy with him in the morning I'll have another look at him."

"Thanks, Doc. Come on b'y. We're going home. No, I'm not carrying you, you big baby! Hold my arm and we'll walk."

They departed, and I took Don and Evelyn upstairs to eat their packed lunches, leaving the outside door open to get rid of the smell.

Next day I did a morning clinic, had a quick lunch and took off home for St. John's. It was a beautiful spring day, sunny and warm, and the miles along the Trans-Canada unrolled in no time. Although the work load was not heavy, I was beat out and had a lot to think about.

Snowstorm

Monday morning, refreshed and relaxed, I headed back, wondering what surprises the next two weeks would bring. The skies were grey and ominous and the highway icy in places, but I arrived without mishap. Evelyn and Don were pleased to see me, and Don carried my suitcase and box of groceries upstairs for me.

As I returned from my weekly visit to South Cove next morning it started to snow heavily. By clinic time at 1:30 ten centimetres were down and it was developing into a full-blown storm. At my suggestion Evelyn and Don both went home. Most of the patients had canceled, anyway. I spent an enjoyable afternoon and evening reading a Dick Francis. The phone never rang once.

Next morning the world was knee-deep in the white stuff. thirty-five centimetres had fallen, blocking the roads and closing the schools. As I stood looking out the front window and drinking my tea, a huge yellow plow chugged along the road and into our parking lot. It made a quick sweep through, essentially clearing it, and returned to the road. I went downstairs and opened the outside door, revealing a drift up to my waist. Pulling on my boots, I collected a shovel from the storeroom, and cleared off the entrance and the area around my car. As I went back indoors the phone was ringing.

"Do you make house calls?" asked an obviously worried woman.

"Yes, but it might be difficult today."

"My old mother has a fever and a cough. She looks real sick, and I don't think she's fit to come out. We have a four-wheel-drive. If we pick you up will you come?"

"Sure," I said, "The plow has just been through here. So, come whenever you can get down."

"Thanks, I think I can hear the plow, now."

The phone rang again. Evelyn. The plow hadn't been down her way yet, but she'd be in as soon as she could. I suggested we do a clinic in the afternoon, if she could get in.

"I called half an hour ago and there was no answer," she said. "I guess you were in the shower?"

"No, I was out shoveling after the plow had been in on its way down the road."

"You don't have to do that!" she exclaimed, shocked.

I said I'd see her later, and we hung up. Don stomped in. The roads weren't too bad, he remarked, as long as you had a four-wheel-drive. I told him about the house call, and he offered to drive me up there in his jeep. He knew the family and where they lived. I made some coffee, and we sat drinking it, and joking about the interesting weather we get in Newfoundland in April. The phone rang again. It was the woman who had called earlier.

"We're plowed out now. OK if we come down for you?"

I checked my house call bag, and arranged with Don that he would answer the phone and give people appointments for the afternoon, until Evelyn arrived.

Andrea, the young woman driving the pickup, was small and pixie-like, and didn't look old enough to have a driver's license. She maneuvered the big machine up hill and down for ten kilometres. At the top of a steep hill she turned off between the trees, and drew up beside a bungalow. It had become mild and the roads were wet and slushy. Even in the fog and drizzle it was a beautiful spot, with views across the bay that must have been stupendous on a clear day.

Andrea's grandmother was eighty-four and alert, despite her fever and rapid shallow breathing. She had pneumonia, and I suggested the cottage hospital. She shook her head firmly, and looked at her daughter.

"We can manage," said Andrea's mother, "We'd rather do that."

I agreed, and checked that she was not allergic to penicillin before giving her a shot. Her daughter said she'd call if she got any worse, and would bring her to the clinic next week to be checked.

Andrea and I slithered our way up and down the hills, and were soon back at the clinic, where she picked up her grandmother's prescription from Don. Evelyn had arrived and was busy making appointments. With the clinic closed the previous twenty-four hours, that afternoon was the busiest in the whole locum. twennty-six people came with various problems and needs. It was 6:30 before we locked up and Evelyn and Don could go home.

In the days following the snowstorm, the locum ground on and I got to know the area, and some of the patients, well. Bob Simms came over twice for his Factor VIII injections, and I gave him his chart to keep with his supplies.

Despite all my speculations, I was never able to fully solve the "mysteries" of Dr. Ali's practice. Perhaps the routine check-ups and blood work for the dieting women were only done because of the fee he could claim from MCP. And the acne pill? Could he have had a deal with the drug company? And if so, was it ethical? I couldn't be sure. As for the Salvation Army officer who I suspected might be addicted to painkillers, I never saw him again during the locum. Perhaps he simply had no more kidney stone attacks during that time.

As for the biggest mystery of all, Dr. Ali's disappearance,

the CEO at the Newfoundland Medical Association called me one day with the answer to that. Dr. Ali was setting up practice in St. John's and had no intention of returning to the outports! The CEO had spoken with him, and told him that it was not an honourable way to treat his patients. Dr. Ali had averred that he would advertise the practice, with house, for sale, and that, far from abandoning his patients, he had arranged two months' care for them. He was not at all remorseful about telling his patients lies and deceiving me.

One day a cheque came in the mail for Evelyn. It covered the whole eight weeks she was working for me, and was accompanied by a pink slip. It was the only contact Dr. Ali made.

Don fretted about his business, and decided to stay open for the time being. At least the patients would be able to get their refills. I suggested he talk to Dr. White, the other doctor in the area, but I had no other help to offer.

The last week dragged dreadfully. Business was very slow as the patients drifted away to the cottage hospital or to Dr. White. On the last day I called him about a few people I hoped he would follow up, and reminded him about Bob Simms. He was familiar with him already, having seen him occasionally on his weekends on call. Would I, asked Dr. White, consider doing a locum for him sometime? I agreed, but pointed out that I was booked up till Labour Day.

At last, I packed up my house call bag and suitcase, and said goodbye to Evelyn, and to Don, feeling bad for both of them, and returned home. Several months later I heard that Dr. White had taken a partner, bought the patients' charts from Dr. Ali, and amalgamated the two practices.

The Cottage Hospital

At The End Of The Road

The cottage hospitals of Newfoundland used to be very isolated and, despite the road building and improved helicopter service, some still are. Blizzards and freezing rain storms can bring travel to a halt wherever you live, but fog and ice are rarely a problem in major centres. The tiny scattered coastal communities are frequently enveloped in such thick fog that road travel, even supposing there are roads, is impossible. Even nowadays, a few communities are only accessible by boat.

Most cottage hospitals have between ten and twenty beds, basic lab and X-ray facilities, and a clinic. Staffed by two, sometimes three, doctors, these hospitals do not usually have a heavy workload, but the work can be very challenging. Even if weather conditions allow for air or road transfer to a major centre, the patient may be too ill for the long journey. From time to time cottage hospital doctors are faced with situations that would stretch even a large hospital to its limits - serious injuries or diabetic comas, for example. There is no surgeon or anaesthetist, and occasionally these GPs have to tackle emergency surgery that simply cannot wait.

In the seventies I once spent six weeks at a cottage hospital, the only doctor there. Two of the regular doctors were a married couple and, as was usual, when they went on holiday the Department of Health replaced them with only one locum — me. The day after I arrived the third doctor, a young man from Hungary with an unpronounceable name with no vowels in it, took off to his homeland for two months. His father had been taken ill and subsequently died.

At St. Christopher's, a small community twenty kilometres away, the doctor, an Irishman, operated a busy clinic, sending patients who needed X-rays or admission to us. Ten days after I started work he went to St. John's for a few days, having warned me to expect to see his patients while he was gone. On the way there he was involved in a car accident and seriously hurt. Now my nearest colleague was eighty kilometres away, on the road to St. John's. Also an Irishman, he worked alone and had no hospital.

So there I was at the tip of a long peninsula, on my own and doing the work of four doctors. I was very busy. Almost every night someone had a baby, an asthma attack, or some other crisis that dragged me from my bed. Inevitably, the days were hectic, too, even on the weekend.

That first Sunday produced the usual handful of minor injuries and flu, but most of the day was taken up with a very upset middle-aged woman, who had required psychiatric treatment intermittently for years. At first I hoped she would settle, but it soon became apparent that she would need transfer to St.John's — a five hour drive. After several attempts I at last located the psychiatrist on call in St. John's. He was not familiar with her and, instead of accepting my referral, said he would look at her chart and call me back. For another four hours the nurses and her family coped as best they could, while I dealt with the other patients.

Finally, I called the psychiatrist back and, after being switched from one extension to another three or four times, got to speak to his resident, who knew nothing about the patient. He promptly suggested I send her in and he, at least, would see her, and try and get in touch with her regular psychiatrist. An hour later, with her daughter and a nurse, she left by ambulance.

While I was eating my overdue, and rather dried up, supper one of the nurses joined me, pulled out a chair and sat down. Obviously, she had bad news.

"What's happened? Don't tell me the ambulance has broken down."

"Oh, no," she answered. "I just had a call from St. Christopher's. The customs officer there has just died. Apparently he was fine, but lay down on the chesterfield and died. They're sending someone to pick you up."

"There's no point in that if he's dead," I said, wearily. "There's nothing I can do. Why don't we get the undertaker to pick him up, and bring him here? If it's a sudden death, we'll have to arrange an autopsy in St. John's, anyhow."

"I suppose so, but they said a neighbour had offered, and is already on his way."

"Who were you talking to?"

"I don't know; another neighbour, I think."

As we spoke, there was a squeal of tires as a car turned in to the hospital. It roared up to the main door, its horn tooting madly, and screeched to a stop. The janitor came in and looked at me thoughtfully.

"You expecting a car from St. Christopher's?"

"Yes. It sounds like they're here."

He nodded, clearly uneasy, then went away. In the lobby, a scruffy young man in ragged jeans and T-shirt, with very long, dirty, curly hair was hopping from one foot to the other. He jerked his head to me to accompany him and went outside. I grabbed my house call bag and followed him out to the car. It was very old and rusty. It was obvious that the passenger door was not only a different colour from the rest of the car, but was intended for a different model.

"You best sit on the seat first, then bring your feet in," advised the driver. "There's a hole in the floor right there."

I did as I was bid, and wriggled about until I fit my rather large bottom between what had once been springs. On a small black-and-white TV perched on the dash, a man and a woman were having a shouting match. The engine burst into life. We jerked forward and tore out of the hospital, and round the corner onto the street. No seatbelts in this old rustbucket, of course. I tried to hold onto the seat, then the dash. In the end I braced myself against the dash as we roared through the community and along the narrow, winding road, swinging around bends and spitting gravel in all directions, including through the hole in the floor. I shut my eyes, partly because of the gravel, and prayed, while the TV struggled to make itself heard.

Suddenly, with a scream of tires and a stink of rubber, we stopped dead.

"We're here," announced my chauffeur, "I'll wait here for you; I want to see this program."

A dazed-looking woman came out of the house and beckoned me in.

"Have you come to see my husband? I don't know what took him. He was all right at supper time."

She took me into their sitting room. A dozen people sat and stood quietly about the room. Two teenagers were on their knees, beside the dead man on the chesterfield, weeping . The widow's lips trembled.

"They're our daughters," she explained, shakily.

At my request, everyone else left the room. I checked the patient, to make sure he was indeed dead, then talked to his wife and family. No, they said, he never had a day's illness in his life. What did I think happened? I explained that very likely he'd had a heart attack, but that an autopsy would be necessary, in St. John's, and that I would arrange it. They nodded without speaking, still shocked by the suddenness of it.

A tall, skinny man came quietly into the room.

"I'm the undertaker," he introduced himself. "His brother called me. Will there be an autopsy?"

"Yes. As I don't know the cause of death, I can't sign the death certificate. He hasn't seen a doctor for years, I gather."

The undertaker gave me the form to sign, declaring that I had examined the patient and that he was indeed dead; he offered to transport the remains to St. John's for autopsy. I thanked him, signed the form, said good-bye to the family, and returned to the car, where my driver was still absorbed by the TV. As I wriggled my way between the springs, and put my feet carefully on the floor to avoid the hole, the engine started with a loud bang. I just had time to brace myself on the dash, and shut my eyes, before we shot off back to the hospital.

At last we screamed to a stop, and I opened my eyes to see Mickey Mouse grinning at me from the TV. I thanked the young man and staggered into the hospital, my wobbly knees not wanting to take me up the steps at first. The janitor came to greet me.

"Are you OK?" he asked, anxiously, "I've been worrying about you, ever since I saw who come to pick you up. He's something else, isn't he?"

I agreed weakly, and gratefully accepted a cup of tea.

The Smuggler

A few days later I had a call from the local RCMP. A man in the lock-up had collapsed. Would I go and look at him? I suggested it would be better if they brought him to the hospital. Well, he seemed OK now, and was about to appear in court, if I said he was fit. Also, it was a delicate situation, and they were trying to avoid publicity.

By the time I'd finished inpatient rounds the car was there, a very handsome young Mountie at the wheel. As I tried to buckle up, I found the seatbelt was jammed. Constable Doucette couldn't release it either, so I rode in a police car breaking the law. Who would be charged, I wondered — me or the RCMP?

"Thanks for coming, Doc," Constable Doucette interrupted my thoughts, "This is a bit awkward. You know we made a big haul of tobacco last week? We caught them just as they were transferring the goods from the French boat to a fishing boat. They were in our waters - just - and we brought them all in. Among the four Frenchmen is a prominent businessman, whom we believe to be the head of the organization. Since he's been our guest he's been on a hunger strike. I think he's feeling a bit weak, and that's why he passed out. Ottawa wants everything kept very quiet, to avoid an international incident. Here we are. Come on in."

The longhaired, middle-aged man in jeans and T-shirt did not look like a prominent businessman to me. As he spoke no English, and my French was not much better, Constable Doucette acted as interpreter. No, said the businessman, he had no pain; no, he took no medications and had never collapsed before; yes, he was normally healthy, and felt fine, now.

When I examined him, everything was normal, including his blood pressure. Why hadn't he eaten? I asked him. Didn't he like the food here? He was protesting his arrest, he said, and would not eat until he was released. How long would it take him to die? Between two and three months, I told him. He was amazed. Surely it would only take a week or two? I assured him that it would take much longer than that and suggested he eat normally, or he would end up in the hospital and the publicity would be much worse.

After telling Constable Doucette that the Frenchman was fit to appear in court, if they let him sit during his interrogation, he drove me back to the hospital to start the busy clinic. Later, I heard that the judge remanded the Frenchman in police custody pending further inquiries. Eventually he was returned home in a deal between the French and Canadian governments.

Island Visit

Alternate weeks we did a clinic on a small island offshore. That second Wednesday I was up early, and had made rounds before the helicopter landed in the hospital car park. I climbed aboard along with the pharmacist, Roger.

First we headed to a small community, ten kilometres away, to pick up the public health nurse. As John, the pilot, prepared to land in her garden, he noticed that her car was gone. He hovered for a few moments, then rose up again and went to search for her, hopping up and down to avoid the electrical cables, but otherwise keeping low enough to identify her striking red station wagon. At the school we circled the building, checking the parking lot — much to the interest of the youngsters assembling below. No sign of her. Maybe she was at the nursing home? Up we went again, to miss the church roof, and followed the main street to the onetime convent, now a home for senior citizens. Still no red station wagon.

"We'll have to go without her!" yelled John over the engine noise. I was relieved. All this leaping about like a kangaroo was hard on my stomach, and I was feeling very queasy by this time.

For ten minutes we flew over water, then rocks, then more water and a fairly large rocky island. On the far side of this island John turned back, and I saw the community huddled between a tall cliff and the sea—about sixty houses, a small school, a church, a wharf and half a dozen boats bobbing in the water.

We landed on the wharf and two men came forward, to help carry our various bags and boxes to the nearby church. The smell of seaweed mixed with fish tickled our noses in the light breeze. In the bright, pristine sunlight the cheerfully painted houses and small church looked so picturesque around the tiny harbour. But what was it like in the winter? I wondered.

"Bleak and isolated," said Roger. "You ever done a clinic in a church before? I thought not. There's a little office you can use. I'll set up in the corner over there."

About twenty people were already sitting in the rows of chairs, as if waiting for a service to start. Mrs. Power, a fat, smiling, older lady welcomed me, and took me through to the office. She showed me the filing cabinet containing the charts but, now that my stomach had returned to its normal place, I was more interested in the pot of coffee on the top. As I poured myself a cup, I explained about the public health nurse. Did I have the stuff to give the babies their needles, she asked? I didn't, though I could easily have brought it, if I had known the nurse wasn't coming.

Taking a cup of coffee for Roger, Mrs. Power went into the main body of the church, and announced that the nurse wasn't coming. Two young women with small babies left, and I got on with the remaining patients.

"Will you be going up to see Mrs. Rowe?" my last patient asked. "The doctor usually does. She can't get out, see. It's not far."

Leaving Roger filling prescriptions, I found Mrs. Rowe's chart and went outside. One of the men who had carried our supplies up from the wharf was out there, and readily agreed to show me the way. Taking my bag he walked along the lane for all of two minutes, and stopped at a small bungalow painted a dazzling pink, with beige trim.

"She's my aunt," he explained as he took me in the back door. "Last year she had a stroke and she can't get out now, but she insists on living here on her own, with just her cat. Me and my cousins check her every day, and do chores for her."

The old lady was delighted to see me. It was wonderful to see the women getting to be doctors and lawyers, she said, bright blue eyes twinkling up at me, and about time, too! Watched by the cat, I checked her over and wrote a prescription to renew her medications, and promised to visit her next time I was on the island. Her nephew took the prescription and my bag, and we walked back to the church.

"That cat's some nosy," he remarked. "You can't do a thing but she's right there keeping an eye on you."

"Cats are like that, aren't they?" I said, wondering how my own two were faring, back in St. John's.

There was one more patient, referred by Roger. His refills had run out. As he only needed his blood pressure taken, he was quickly dealt with. Roger refilled his prescription and we packed up.

"We go to Mrs. Power's for dinner," Roger informed me, "She won't let us pay, but I always leave five dollars on the sideboard."

He led me to the last house on the waterfront — about five minutes walk. In the kitchen Mrs. Power, still smiling, was busy creating delicious aromas.

"It's salt beef and cabbage," she said, "I hope you like Newfoundland food."

"That's great," I told her. "I don't need to worry about my allergy to shellfish."

"I can't eat lobster or crab. They make me break out," she said. "You got that, too? I hope you're not allergic to cats. I got five here now."

"No, I like cats. I've got two of my own back in St. John's."

"What do you do when you're away like this?"

"My tenant in the apartment upstairs looks after them for me."

"You wouldn't like any more, would you? I've got three kittens to find homes for. How about you, Roger?"

He shook his head, and led me into the sitting room where John, the pilot, sat in an armchair with a cat on his lap. Three delightful kittens chased each other about the room.

"Everybody here has cats," commented Roger, dropping onto the chesterfield. "I think there's more cats than people on this island."

"No mice or rats, though, " said Mrs. Power from the doorway. "Coffee or tea, Doctor?"

I opted for tea, put my five dollars on the sideboard among the family photos, and went to look out the window. From this slightly raised vantage point, I could see the whole community in front and to the right of me, protected by the towering cliff behind it. To the left the sea sparkled a brilliant blue-green, and seagulls swooped down on a small boat chugging in. Over our delicious dinner I asked Mrs. Power if she lived there alone.

"Oh, yes," she replied. "My man was lost at sea eighteen year ago. The children were small then. One of my boys is still here, fishing. The two girls are in St. John's. They're all married, but my younger boy isn't yet. He's in the Armed Forces, in New Brunswick."

"It can't have been easy," I said.

"No, but they've done good, and I'm proud of them. But I don't see much of them, or my grandchildren, except for Andrew and his crowd. I see them every day."

On the short flight back I was marveling at the panorama of sea, sky and rocks when, suddenly, the door beside me swung open, and I had an uninterrupted view from my feet to the rocks way below. Terrified, I turned to John, and tried to grab on to his seat. He pointed at my seatbelt, and I realized that I was safely buckled up, and there was no need for panic. To my astonishment, Roger, behind me, calmly unbuckled, stood up and leaned out, and closed the door.

Minutes later, on solid ground at the hospital car park, I was still shaking, but he just shrugged his shoulders nonchalantly, and went on home. As soon as my jellified legs would walk properly, I went on into the hospital to do another clinic. One of the pharmaceutical reps had been in and left me some samples, and my mail which he had kindly picked up at my house before leaving St. John's the previous day. He would phone me in the evening.

Emergency at the Lighthouse

The following week, the lightkeeper at another of the outlying islands was taken ill. John was already occupied, so another helicopter was called in from Gander. The pilot had no difficulty landing by the lighthouse and picking up the sick man. But he was not familiar with our little town, and buzzed around overhead trying to decide which building was the hospital. Although the ambulance was parked nearby, and the ambulance driver, the janitor, a nurse and me were all standing on the steps waving frantically, he chose a building just down the street. It was the school. The nurse and I jumped into the ambulance with Pat, the driver, and hurried down.

Beside the now-quiet chopper Mrs. Walsh, the principal, stood talking to the pilot. Dozens of eager faces lined the windows, and two or three of the older children came outside.

"Stay indoors," ordered the principal, waving her hands at them. "Everybody is to stay indoors."

"Guess I goofed," said the young, but very bald, pilot, grinning at us. "This poor fellow is in some misery, I tell you."

He looked at Pat. "Are you going to see him here, Doctor?"

"I'm the ambulance driver. This is the doctor," said Pat, nodding at me.

"You were expecting a man doctor, weren't you?" Mrs Walsh teased him.

He nodded sheepishly, and opened the door and assisted me and the nurse up into the helicopter. It was apparent that the poor lightkeeper was having a gall bladder attack, and would need to go on to St.John's. I sent Pat back to the hospital for some medication and syringes while I wrote a note for the Health Sciences Centre, on the back of a pad of itinerary forms produced by the pilot. The nurse gave the patient a shot; the pilot started the engine. Blades whirring, the chopper lifted high above the school, as the children all came tumbling out to watch it. Pat and the nurse returned to the hospital, while I stopped to explain the situation to Mrs. Walsh and answer questions fired at me by the excited youngsters.

"Not much work will get done today," commented Mrs. Walsh. "I think I'll have the younger ones draw pictures of this event. They'll enjoy that."

"Bring the pictures over to the hospital, and we could pin them up in the waiting room," I offered.

"I will. They'll love that. Thanks."

She went indoors and I hurried back to the hospital to phone St. John's.

The waiting room was already decorated with pictures drawn by the local schoolchildren, but they were getting tatty. The exhibit titled "Going to the Hospital" had attracted an enthusiastic response. One, beside my office door, was particularly striking. Created by an eight-year-old asthmatic, a regular "customer," it showed a tiny person in a tiny bed, with a large adult holding a huge syringe and needle, looming over her. Another showed a minute figure in the bottom left hand corner. The rest of the paper was covered with a black "box", presumably the X-ray machine. All these should be kept, I thought, but it would be great to get some new pictures up.

By the end of my six weeks I was exhausted. When the couple I was replacing returned, they were shocked to find that I had been alone all that time, and that the Department of Health had not appointed a locum for the Hungarian doctor, nor for the Irishman at St.Christopher's. At their instigation I wrote to the Department, pointing out that I had been doing the work of four doctors, and being paid for only one, and requesting remuneration accordingly. After further correspondence, and several months delay, they gave me "chief medical officer" pay, instead of "assistant medical officer," and refunded deductions made for my board and lodging.

The Power Outage

Glitter Storm

On April 1984 the easternmost part of Newfoundland was hit by a "glitter" storm. The freezing rain fell for hours and hours, as layers of ice built up on trees and power lines. Cars and buildings became encapsulated in thick ice. Roads and sidewalks turned into skating rinks.

But the hardest part was losing the power. Under the weight of several inches of ice, power and phone lines fell, sometimes snapping off but more often bringing poles and pylons crashing down with them. People with propane stoves and kerosene heaters suddenly became very popular with their neighbours. Stores did a tremendous business in candles and flashlights. organizations like the Salvation Army fed thousands of people that weekend, cooking vast pots of soup on gas stoves.

On the Monday I started a three week locum on a nearby island. The grey clouds hung so low it was still almost dark, as I hammered and scraped at the "tarpaulin" of ice completely covering my car. Then the doors would not open — none of them. I crept and skidded up the ice-covered steps into the house, and grabbed the box of matches off the kitchen table. The candle there, my only source of heat and light for three days, was now only an inch tall. Tonight I would be in the dark, as I knew all the stores in St. John's were cleaned out of them.

Four matches and a burned finger and thumb later I finally got into the car, started the engine and slithered out of the driveway onto the ice and dirt on the street. Outside the city the roadsides were strewn with broken cables, and the trees doubled right over with the weight of the ice. Rocks shone spookily in the feeble light. By the time I arrived at the ferry terminal I was warmer than I had been for three days. It was tempting to stay in the cozy car, but the boat was there waiting.

Gingerly, with tiny steps, I inched my way down to the slippery wharf. Passing my house call bag to a helpful boatman, I scrambled aboard behind a small oriental man, who was obviously well-known to the crew. Remembering that one of the doctors on the island was from the Philippines, I introduced myself to him. He shook hands and offered to share the taxi that would meet him on the far side.

The island had been very hard hit by the storm, Carlos told me as we chugged our way across the tickle; chunks of ice clanging loudly against the sides of the boat. Everybody had lost their power and their phones. It had been necessary to admit numerous elderly and disabled people to the hospital, which had its own generator. The hospital, he continued, had been built when the mines were active, and the population much larger. When he left for home on Friday evening it was full for the first time in years.

"Who is looking after the patients, then?" I asked.

"The third doctor," said Carlos. "He's a young Irishman called Mick O'Brien."

"I expect he has been very busy."

The twenty minute ride was over. Carlos led the way to a waiting taxi and introduced me to the driver. As we drove away the first of four Newfoundland Power trucks lumbered off the ferry and up the ramp.

In spite of Carlos' account, I was stunned by the devastation. Heaped up cables, tree branches, and the occasional transformer littered the streets and gardens. The utility poles, sheathed in ice, had snapped off about halfway down; the remnants stood starkly against the sky as we crested a small hill. Everything was smothered in the thick ice, which glowed eerily as the sun tried half-heartedly to emerge through the clouds.

"How did you get on over the weekend?" Carlos asked the driver.

"It's been hard, and it's going to last a while. We got no water, see, except at the hospital. The pump at the reservoir's electric," he added, in answer to my startled glance. "We're supposed to be getting power and phone people from all over today. I see there was four rigs on the ferry you come on."

"Yes," I said, "and there's several more on the other side, waiting for the next boat."

"It's getting enough poles that will be the problem," said the taxi driver. "Every single one is broke right off. We need dozens, no, hundreds of them."

At the hospital Carlos led me through the waiting area and around to the cafeteria, where he introduced me to two nurses and three members of the kitchen staff.

"Dr. O'Brien about anywhere, do you know?" he asked them.

"He's on the floor," replied one of the nurses, as she prepared to depart. "I'll tell him you're here. You all going to make rounds when you had your coffee?"

We promised to do so. Mick O'Brien soon joined us. Tall, skinny and red-haired, he looked too young to be out of high school, let alone medical school. He smiled shyly.

"It's good to see you. It's been like a war zone here."

"Outside it looks like nuclear winter," said Carlos. "Were you very busy?"

"Not me, really, mostly the nurses. The patients' relatives have been helping a lot. Of course, it's nice and warm here, and we have water. The people can't even flush their toilets, and there's not enough snow left for them to use that. Besides, most have no means of melting it. Oh, here's Smudge."

Smudge?

"Your secretary," explained Carlos.

Smudge, about thirty-five, with thick glasses and an attractive smile, came over to the table and introduced herself while Mick got her a coffee.

"It's awful at the office," she complained, running a hand through her dark, very curly hair. "No heat, no light, no water, no phone. A few people have been in, and I told them you'd do a clinic this afternoon. Is that OK?"

I nodded. It was only ten o'clock, but there were inpatients to see with Carlos and Mick.

"I'll put a notice in the window that you'll be there from one to four. It will have to be a walk-in clinic as the phones are out."

Two Mounties entered the cafeteria, picked up some coffee, and joined us. One put a walkie-talkie on the table.

"There's one of these at the nurses' desk, and another at the Town Hall," he said. "If you need anything call us on them. We have another radio at the office we can use to call the RCMP in St. John's. The phone people are hoping to get a line in, at least to the hospital, in the next couple of days."

We three doctors finished our coffee and went round to the ward. The nurses were run off their feet with the huge influx of patients, so we took the cart with the charts on and made rounds on our own. Mick was familiar with all the patients and told us about them. By the time we had seen them all, and Mick had shown me the rest of the hospital, it was lunchtime. Carlos, on call that day, had long since disappeared to the Emergency Department to deal with a few problems there.

As we tucked into liver and onions Mick chatted away. He had only been in Newfoundland three months, and was finding it "very interesting," and quite different from his home town, Dublin.

"The work here is so varied, you couldn't possibly be bored, and the people are so friendly and kind."

I agreed and told him that even after nearly twenty years in Newfoundland, I still felt the same way about it.

The Office

Outside, the temperature had noticeably increased. Underfoot it was still slippery, but getting slushy too, and I slid my way carefully across the hospital car park, and down the main street to the office. Ice falling off the trees tinkled and crashed about me like breaking glass. On the other side of the street a large sheet of ice growled off the roof of a house and smashed onto the sidewalk below. Fortunately, nobody was underneath.

In the office, which had once been a butcher's shop ("still is" one wag said to me) two men in coveralls were wrestling with a sheet, trying to make a screen for the waiting area.

"Hello, you the doctor?" asked one.

I introduced myself.

"I'm Dennis, Smudge's husband, and this is my brother, Gordon. There are no windows in your rooms, so we figured you'd best see patients in here, where you get some light. People won't mind waiting in the dark. So we moved the chairs in there and hauled the bed out here. That OK?"

I thanked them and asked where Smudge was.

"Gone to her Dad's to borrow a lantern, so she can at least write in the book and find the patients charts for you. Dr.Gosse chose a good week to go to Florida, didn't he?"

"You bet he did! Why is she called Smudge?"

"I don't know, but she's been called Smudge ever since she were a baby. Her right name is Eudora Mildred. I didn't know that until our wedding, when the priest called her Eudora Mildred! I'd never thought of her as anything but

Smudge." He laughed. "I was so surprised I nearly messed up me lines."

A young woman with a small girl came in the door.

"Is the doctor coming, Dennis?"

He indicated me. "She's here."

"Oh, can you have a look at Sherry? She's got a real bad cold. I don't wonder at it either. This is terrible! Did you ever see the like of it? You got water here?"

Dennis shook his head. I gave her a chair and asked her to wait for Smudge's return. She sat Sherry on her lap and sang to her, while I gave Dennis and Gordon a hand with the sheet. Soon we had it rigged up, so that people coming in the door could walk up to Smudge's desk and on into the pitch-dark waiting area without seeing into the makeshift examining room.

"You going to see the patients in here, then?" asked Sherry's mother.

"It's the only place with windows," explained Dennis, "so folks will have to wait in the dark, then get seen out here. Them venetian blinds will stop them lookin' in. We'll have to make do. The whole island is cleaned right out of candles, batteries and that."

"So is St. John's," I said, closing the blind in the corner where the examining table stood, and leaving the other two open. Despite the grey, cloudy day the light was fairly good.

Smudge returned with an elderly man, her father, who carried an oldfashioned lantern. He placed it on Smudge's desk in the far corner and lit it. Then he climbed onto Smudge's chair, removed a spider plant from a hook in the ceiling, and hung the lantern there. It cast a flickering orange glow on the walls, the chart racks and Smudge's desk, but it was a big improvement on the previous gloom.

"Is it Halloween?" asked Sherry, wide-eyed.

Smudge's father, husband and brother-in-law departed. She passed me Sherry's chart, and I examined her without undressing her, just fiddling my stethoscope under her clothes. It was too cold for any of us to take even our coats off.

"What about the drugstore?" I asked Smudge.

"He's open this afternoon. I told him I'd stop by on my way home to tell him you'd finished the clinic. It's some hard without a phone!"

Throughout the afternoon patients came in ones and twos, apologizing for their dirty state, and for not making appointments. Neither mattered, as I said a dozen times; it just couldn't be helped.

The last patient was a middle-aged man for a blood pressure check.

"You bring your car over here?" he asked me.

"No," I replied, puzzled, "I left it on the other side."

"Good thing. The wind's gone around, and the ice just come right in. The tickle is packed with it. God knows when the ferry will run again. It sure can't get through that lot."

"How will people get back and forth?"

"Helicopter. If you can afford it! It's not right, them making a fortune out of us because of the ice. Good job we got the kids off yesterday."

"Where did they go?"

"Me brother's. Lots of people done that, especially us with older ones. It'll be weeks before the schools reopen here, but St. John's should be back to normal in a day or two."

"I don't know about that," I protested, "There was still no power when I left this morning."

"It's back on, most parts of St. John's. It was on the radio."

He went on and, at Smudge's suggestion, she and I went over to the hospital for a cup of tea. The administrator joined us and introduced herself to me. If I wanted to stay anytime, she said, there was room in the staff quarters. I thanked her and said that I had to go home that night, as I had a meeting that, as far as I knew, had not been canceled. Also, I was concerned about my house and two cats. Smudge drove me to the wharf where the ferry sat idle. On the far side I could see two more Power trucks waiting.

"They won't get over here for days. Even the icebreaker won't be able to clear this lot," said Smudge, "The helicopter can only take four at a time. You might as well stay in the car and keep warm, until your turn."

Huge pieces of ice, some as big as small houses, were jammed solidly into the narrow tickle. The helicopter buzzed back and forth. On the fourth trip my turn came, and I climbed aboard with three men from Newfoundland Power. $20 for the four minute ride! I decided that, while the ice was in, I would stay at the hospital all week, and only go home on the weekends. My tenant upstairs could look after the cats and the house, as he did so often when I was away on locums.

Most of the trees were now standing more or less upright, and the rocks no longer shone with ice, but the drive home was dreary. As I opened my back door a rush of warm air welcomed me. The power was on! The cats glanced up from their favourite sleeping place, the shelf over the radiator in the dining room, now nice and warm again. My tenant came downstairs.

"Isn't this wonderful!" He spread his arms wide. "Warmth and light! Your meeting's canceled, by the way. They called just now. I'm making supper. Come up in about half an hour."

Later, over delicious curry, I told him about my day, and the helicopter. He willingly agreed to feed the cats, so that I could save $40 a day.

Back To The Island

Next morning it was raining lightly as I drove to the ferry terminal. A raw wind blew off the ice, still packed in solid, weird-shaped heaps in the tickle. The big rigs parked there the previous night had gone, dispatched to other areas until the ferry operated again. About twenty men in vivid orange coveralls and bright yellow hard hats, were ahead of me waiting for the helicopter. Why didn't they lay on another helicopter, or a bigger one? the man in front of me wondered.

"You work for Newfoundland Power?" he asked me.

"No, I work at the hospital."

The pilot, just returned, scowled at me.

"My instructions are to give the Power people priority, and everyone else got to wait," he stated firmly. "The other doctors will have to manage without you for a bit longer."

"That's OK. Do I get a discount for waiting?"

"Are you kidding? My boss would have my head!"

"Is it expensive?" inquired one of the Power men. "We're not paying, of course."

"It's twenty dollars for the four minute ride," I told him. "The ferry is only two dollars."

His jaw dropped. "That's a rip-off!"

A middle-aged man in a smart suit, and carrying a briefcase, joined us. He was from the Department of Energy, Mines and Resources, he grandly told the pilot, and would thank him to put him on the next flight. The pilot refused, saying that power and phone men had priority. The government man became very annoyed, and demanded to go next. A muttering ran along the dozen workmen still lined up. One pointed at me.

"She's a DOCTOR!" he informed him, "and she's waiting. Don't you tell the pilot you'll report him. He'll report you more likely."

The man gave up and took his place behind me, grumbling to himself. When my turn came, an hour later, I was the fourth person on. So he, with his fancy briefcase, was left standing on the wharf all alone. As we took off we all waved enthusiastically, but he didn't even smile.

At the far side I went into the ferry office to phone for a taxi. The ticket clerk who, of course, was doing nothing at all, recognized me and stubbed out his cigarette, locked the office and kindly drove me to the hospital in his car.

"Does the ice usually get this bad?" I asked him. Though I had lived in St. John's for years, I had never taken much notice of the ice "around the bay."

"No," he replied, "this is real bad. But we always get some. The icebreaker comes and gets the ferry moving again. But even the icebreaker can't deal with this."

It was almost ten o'clock, so I went straight round to the nurses' desk. Mick and Carlos were just finishing rounds.

"You sleep in this morning?" asked Carlos, with a grin.

"No, I had to wait an hour for my turn on the chopper. The Power men had priority." I told them about the government man and we all had a good laugh.

"Are you on call today?" one of the nurses asked me.

"Yes," I confessed. "Is anything happening?"

"There's two people in Emergency. They haven't been there long. one has a cut needs suturing and the other's hurt her ankle."

I dealt with these, then joined the two men in the cafeteria for a welcome cup of coffee. Carlos told me of a patient of Dr. Gosse's he had admitted the previous evening, with emphysema. He was much better this morning, but would I take him over? I agreed to do so.

The young woman with the injured ankle hobbled in and passed me her X-rays. Holding them up to the strip lighting overhead, I checked them carefully. No fractures, I was able to assure her. I gave them back to her, and told her to take them to Emergency and have a bandage put on. She looked at me wistfully.

"Can I wash my hair while I'm here? It's driving me mad."

"I'm sorry," I sympathized. "The administrator decided that nobody, except inpatients and staff, would be allowed showers. This could go on for weeks."

She limped off, and Carlos and I returned to the floor to see the man with emphysema. Then Carlos showed me the doctors' quarters. A suite with its own kitchen and bathroom, originally intended for the doctor-in-charge, was occupied by

Mick. Carlos, like me, lived in St. John's, and usually only stayed over when he was on call, using one of the two bedrooms off a small sitting room. While the ferry was tied up we would both stay all week, and go home on the weekends.

The week wore on, not particularly busy. The power men and the phone men (over 100 all told) worked from "can see to can't see" in the intermittent rain and raw northeast wind. One of the schools was opened and they bunked there, getting their meals at a church hall equipped with gas stoves. The local people were kept busy cooking for them, fetching water from the hospital, and simply surviving.

All of them had relatives in St. John's, and most had sent their children over on Monday morning, when the ferry was still running. Reluctant to abandon their homes in the crisis, most of the adults, and the small kids, remained on the island, struggling to cope without water, heat or light. Fridges and freezers weren't working, naturally, and piles of food were given to feed the workmen, before it spoiled. The supermarket and the smaller stores were cleaned out in a couple of days.

The hospital's emergency generator, not designed to operate full tilt for days on end, started coughing. The lights would fade, and everyone stop what they were doing and hold their breath anxiously. Then it got going again; everything brightened and we all heaved a sigh of relief. The two maintenance men stayed with it day and night, coaxing it, swearing at it, adjusting this and that, and somehow keeping it running for ten days.

On Thursday that first week they got a phone line into the hospital, the school and church hall the workmen were using, the Town Hall, the RCMP, and the clinic. At Smudge's suggestion the people were allowed to use the clinic phone to touch base with their children in St. John's (a local call). Each afternoon I arrived at the clinic to find the dark waiting area full of people, many just standing round propping up the walls. My heart would sink at the prospect of such a busy clinic, but most were waiting their turn to use the phone. All were very cooperative and didn't talk long; they were extremely grateful for the service.

Friday afternoon Mick and Carlos left for St. John's. At my instigation they finished early, to avoid a long wait for the helicopter. I gave Mick the keys to my car and house, and a note for my tenant. Mick hadn't been off the island for nearly a month, and badly needed a weekend away.

Labour Pains and Tonsils

The sun was shining brilliantly as I walked back to the hospital after the clinic. To my right, great masses of glittering and winking ice creaked and growled. Ahead they stretched to the horizon, broken only by the red slash of the icebreaker, sitting helpless a mile or so away. The cliffs on the far side of the tickle, normally brown but now sheeted with ice, towered behind it. The biting wind soon drove me indoors.

That evening a girl of fifteen presented in early labour. Very tiny, she might need a caesarian section, and was booked for St.Clare's. Time to call the helicopter. The nurse on duty called the emergency number to arrange it. There were none available, she was told. It would mean bringing one in from Gander. Realizing she was having difficulty persuading the man on the other end that this was not only necessary but urgent, I took the phone.

It was the only time I had problems getting a helicopter. Always, they would locate one somewhere and send it on its way. This fellow was totally uninterested in our dilemma. All the helicopters were busy, he insisted doggedly, he couldn't do anything about it. But what were they all doing at 10:00 P.M? I asked. He couldn't say. Then I remembered the icebreaker.

"There must be a chopper on the icebreaker," I pointed out.

Well, he wouldn't know about that. Furious and frustrated, I called the Coast Guard direct. Of course there was a helicopter on the icebreaker, said the officer on duty, but it was too small for a stretcher case. No matter, I told him. The girl could sit up.

Fifteen minutes later the helicopter landed in the hospital car park, and the girl and her mother were helped aboard. An ambulance would meet them at the Health Sciences Centre for transport to St.Clare's. I returned to the hospital to find the Director of Nursing awaiting me. She smiled.

"The nurses called me, as they always do when anything unusual crops up. What a to-do! Thank goodness you knew how to handle it. If Mick had been on, he would have been stuck."

"That idiot couldn't have cared less," I said, crossly. "I've never had anything like it before. They always do their darnedest to help."

"We should lodge a complaint about him," she suggested. "We'll talk to the administrator on Monday morning, both of us if that's OK with you."

Saturday morning we had a call from St. Clare's. The girl had had a normal, though not easy delivery and was doing well.

The next twenty-four hours were very quiet, with just the occasional patient. All the chronically sick and frail were in the hospital already, and nearly half the island's population remained in St. John's. People who had gone to work by ferry as usual on Monday morning were still there, as were most of the teenagers and university students.

Phone and power workers battled on, their heavy, waterproof boots helping them stay upright in the icy mud. It was their hands that took a beating. Frequently having to remove their thick gloves to perform a more delicate task, many men developed severe chapping with raw, bleeding areas on their knuckles. Four appeared on Saturday evening to see what I could do for them. I gave them a jar of the ointment we used for bedsores, and handed each of them a pair of plastic disposable gloves.

"When you go to bed, put it on the raw places fairly thickly," I instructed them. "Then put the gloves on, so you don't lose it on the blankets."

"Some of the other fellows got the same trouble," said one. "Should we give this stuff to them, too?"

"Sure." I passed him the box of gloves and they left.

On Sunday afternoon the wind was blowing harder than ever, and cold rain poured down, sometimes mixed with snow. A large phone company rig with two "cherrypickers" up behind pulled into the car park, coming to a halt right outside the door. Two burly men jumped out and turned to help a third, almost lifting him down from the high cab. Taking a nearby wheelchair I went out to them. They sat him in it and we all went indoors.

"What happened?" I asked, thinking he had had an accident.

"He's real sick," said one. "Can't stop shivering and can't hardly walk. This morning he didn't look too good, and didn't eat his breakfast. I asked him if he was sick, but he said he was OK."

The patient drooped in the chair, his teeth chattering.

"I got the flu," he whispered.

"Guess you got a sore throat, too, have you?" I asked, removing his hard hat to get a better look at him.

"Can't swallow."

A nurse from the floor arrived as the two men were helping him out of his heavy, wet coveralls. She glanced at him, then at me.

"You going to admit him?"

"I'll have to. He can't bunk down at the school in this state. Can we put him straight into a bed?"

"There's just the one in the corridor, but it will have to do."

The two men went back to their work, and the nurse

wheeled the patient round to the floor, where we put him into a johnny shirt, and into bed.

His lips were chapped and dry, and speech and swallowing were obviously very painful, but he managed to tell us that his name was Barry Oldford and that he was from Grand Falls. I examined his mouth expecting to see a bad case of tonsillitis, but his whole throat was flaming red, with dark areas where his tonsils should have been.

"Did you have your tonsils out recently?"

"Ten days ago."

"You shouldn't be working, especially outdoors in the cold and rain, so soon!"

"I know, but I felt good, see, so I come. I was OK until last night.'

Examining him more thoroughly I found he was moderately dehydrated, had a high fever and noises in his chest, implying pneumonia. Despite his intravenous, and being in the busy corridor, he slept right through the night.

Food and Water

As most of the workmen had stayed on the island all weekend, Mick and Carlos didn't have to wait long for the helicopter on Monday morning, and walked into the hospital together just before nine. We made rounds of all the inpatients, including the only new one, young Barry Oldford. After nearly twenty-four hours of intravenous fluids and medications, he was much better, though still having difficulty talking and swallowing.

"When can I go back to work?" he whispered.

"Not for at least two weeks," I replied, fighting the urge to whisper back. "In a few days we'll let you out of here and you can go home. Then it will be up to your own doctor."

"I was hoping to get lots of overtime," he admitted, ruefully. "I'm getting married in June, see, and we want to buy a house."

A male attendant came with a wheelchair and took him for a chest X-ray. We doctors went to the cafeteria, where Mick passed me a bundle of mail and chatted about his weekend. He had thoroughly enjoyed himself doing nothing much. My tenant had taken him to a party with the "folk arts" crowd, where he had been persuaded to play the fiddle. I told them about the problems over the chopper on Friday night. Carlos was surprised. Like me, he had never experienced any difficulties.

The cook came across to our table.

"There's only sandwiches for lunch," she reported, "and I don't know what we'll do for supper, even for the patients. Usually we have plenty, but with so many more, and the ferry not running, we're just about out. Everybody's the same. There's no food anywhere."

"But what about the workmen?" cried Carlos.

She shook her head. "I don't know. The mayor was trying to get an airlift of food last week, but the government didn't do anything."

"Surely they'll do something now!" I insisted. "We've been on the national news every day for the last week. They must know that the stores are cleaned out, and fridges and freezers not functioning. Besides, people gave all they had to feed the workmen."

A small plane flew overhead.

"Maybe that's food," said Mick, hopefully. He had a teenager's appetite.

"Huh, more likely some government fat cat come to see if we need it," said the cook, tartly, going to the serving area as more staff came in looking for coffee.

But it was food, flown in by Newfoundland Power for their workmen. The plane returned twice more. The second load was brought to the hospital and the third taken to the Town Hall, where council members doled it out.

As the taxi driver had predicted, the chief problem with restoring power was obtaining enough poles. Fortunately, a large number had been brought over on the Monday morning, before the ice closed in. Mick had noticed a huge pile, about a hundred he thought, sitting at the terminal on the far side, waiting for the ferry to run again. Power and phone lines were temporarily attached to the sides of buildings or trees until more poles arrived.

That Tuesday morning Newfoundland Power got a line out to the reservoir and got the pump going. Arriving at the office early, I was surprised to see Smudge leaping and dancing around the waiting room.

"We've got water! We've got water!" she sang. Seeing me she stopped, embarrassed.

"Is it really on again?" I asked eagerly.

"Just us, the Town Hall, the hospital and the school/bunkhouse at the moment. The town engineers are working as hard as they can to get the airlocks out of the system."

Two men walked in, each carrying two buckets.

"You got water, Smudge?" pleaded one.

"Help yourselves," she offered.

"Don't drink it for the time being," I begged them. "Just use it to flush your toilets. It's bound to be full of germs at first. Tell everyone not to drink it."

They filled their buckets and departed. I phoned the administrator at the hospital, and she agreed to arrange the necessary lab tests. Then I called the mayor, and told him to put up notices, and to tell everybody that the water would not be fit to drink at first. Amazingly, we had got through the ten days without an intestinal epidemic, I said, and it would be a shame if it happened now. He pointed out that the water was "kinda dirty looking" and he thought people would be sensible.

By Wednesday night everyone in the town had water. On Thursday the smaller communities were hooked up too.

On Wednesday afternoon, when I was on call again, one of the young workmen presented with a pain in his side and throwing up. Even without the blood work it was clear he had appendicitis. His supervisor was with him, and agreed to arrange for someone to meet the chopper on the far side and transport him to one of the St. John's hospitals

Late that night an elderly man was brought in after suffering a severe stroke. Several family members sat with him for the next few hours as he quietly died.

A major nuisance at the hospital after the first week was that we ran out of garbage bags. For medical waste we took down a tatty shower curtain and made two garbage bags out of it. We had almost finished stapling the sides together when we ran out of staples for the second time. No more staples anywhere in the hospital. The administrator managed to scrounge some from the RCMP.

That Thursday evening, as we ate our supper in the cafeteria, one of the janitors strode in carrying a box.

"Look what I found in the linen cupboard! Sixty garbage bags."

"I bet you're GLAD," remarked a male attendant.

The janitor was known as "The Man from Glad" for several days.

Fog and Ice

By Thursday I was really looking forward to the weekend. With the water on and the airlifts of food, things had improved considerably, but life still wasn't easy. The hospital was choc-a-bloc with the chronically ill, and the people still had no power and no phones at their homes. The wind blew steadily from the northeast, keeping the ice piled right into the tickle. The icebreaker had freed itself and moved down the bay to wait patiently for the wind to change.

Friday morning we awoke to thick fog. The hospital seemed to be marooned on an island of its own. With no street lights the rest of the world was invisible. The wind had dropped, leaving an eerie silence broken only by the occasional creak from the ice offshore.

"It doesn't look as if you'll be home for the weekend, after all," said Carlos at breakfast. "I'm on call, so I hope we don't have any serious emergencies. We're completely cut off now."

"Maybe it will lift this afternoon," I said optimistically.

"You've lived in Newfoundland too long to believe that!" retorted Carlos.

After rounds and coffee all three of us went outside. It was much milder and completely calm. We jumped at a loud crack away to our left, followed by a thunderous boom.

"The ice is moving!" cried a lab technician who had joined us. "Sometimes it goes all at once, if the wind goes around. Not much will happen on a day like this though."

"Maybe the icebreaker will make it now," suggested Mick.

"Dare say it will try again now," agreed the lab technician.

Later, I strolled over to the clinic in the gloom. Out in the tickle I could hear the rumble of the icebreaker's engines, and the creaks and groans of the ice as the ship tried to batter its way through it.

"You won't get home today," said Smudge sympathetically. "Do you think you can stand it?"

"I suppose so. Worse things have happened to me," I replied wearily. "But I wish I'd brought more books to read."

"My sister's the librarian," said Smudge. "The library's closed, of course, but she'd take you over to pick some out. You'll need them seeing as you're not on call."

I cheered up immediately, and arranged to meet Smudge's sister after the clinic. She resembled Smudge so much I wondered if they were twins. But not so. Smudge was two years older, said Barbara. We walked to the library, and I soon chose four books by flashlight. I promised to leave them with Smudge when I'd finished with them.

Saturday lunchtime the news flew around the hospital. The icebreaker had got through, and the ferry was going to try and make a crossing. No passengers except some workmen. If they made it they would load up the remaining poles and return. Leaving Carlos at the hospital, Mick and I borrowed a car and drove to the wharf. The icebreaker, which had looked so small and helpless out in the bay, now loomed huge and scarlet, through the fog. Two men with large axes were leaping about on the ice trying to chop the ferry free.

"Boy! That's dangerous work," muttered Mick, staring at them in astonishment.

The ferry engines roared as they tried to charge through the remaining ice. On the second go they made it, and the two men climbed back onto the wharf. They went into the ticket office and locked the axes away again. In the next few minutes first the breaker, then the ferry, vanished into the fog. The noise of their engines echoed back and forth, punctuated by thuds and clangs as the ice moved. It was dark when they returned. The crossing, usually twenty minutes, had taken an hour and a half going, and two hours coming back.

Sunday the fog lifted a little. The ferry made another crossing, assisted by the icebreaker, and picked up drums of electric and phone cable and other supplies.

That final week of my locum was much easier, as the power and phones were gradually restored. The ferry, led by the icebreaker, was able to make limited trips. The sun was out and a light breeze blew from the south on Friday afternoon, when I took leave of Mick, the hospital staff and Smudge— taking care to return the library books. As Smudge drove Carlos and me to the ferry I thanked her for all her help and support. She smiled.

"Come again in the summer. It's beautiful here then," she invited me.

The tickle was still full of ice, but it had loosened up, and the ferry shoved its way through without difficulty. The icebreaker was nowhere in sight.

"It's gone to Botwood," volunteered a crew member. "They've got heavy ice there too. I hopes the wind don't change again, or this lot will come right back in."

In no time I was home. Life in St. John's had long since

returned to normal. The island could have been on the other side of the globe.

House Calls

For the patients the benefits of house calls are obvious, but for the doctor they are a mixed blessing. Seeing the patient at home gives you new insights into the disease or disability, and the effect it has on the patient, the family and, sometimes, the community. Examining the patient on a low bed, with poor lighting and no privacy, can be less than satisfactory, however. Dogs and small children are apt to misinterpret your motives and rush to the patient's defense. House calls are also time-consuming and not very lucrative.

But, without question, the hardest thing about the house call is finding the place, especially rural areas like the small Newfoundland outports where I worked as a locum. Communities often refrain from identifying themselves, streets are not named or not labeled, and there are few landmarks and no numbers on the houses. Directions from anxious relatives may be inadequate, inaccurate or downright misleading.

Responding to a request to visit an elderly man, I proceeded to "The Legion" and turned left just past it. The tiny lane terminated in a cluster of houses, four of them bungalows, but none painted cream with green trim. Nobody was about, of course, and I had just decided to go to the nearest one and ask, when a sign on its neighbour caught my eye. It said "No Smoking, Oxygen in Use." So I went there and it was the right one.

"You did say it was cream with green trim, didn't you?" I asked the patient's wife.

"Yes," she replied, then, "Oh, my! We painted it last time Bill was in hospital, so the smell wouldn't bother him. I forgot about that."

She went outside and looked at her house, painted blue with white trim, as if seeing it for the first time.

Another time, I was told the house was on the main road, the third house on the right after the United Church. It sounded simple enough but, on my arriving there, the startled occupant directed me to the next house along. When I questioned the caller about it, she told me the second house didn't count, because there was nobody living in it!

While I was examining the patient, we were all startled by the scream of a siren close by. An ambulance pulled into the driveway, so I went out to see what was happening. The driver jumped out and came over to me. Normally neat and tidy, he was covered in dirt and blood and was quite upset.

"I saw your car and pulled in here," he said. "He's lost some load of blood, I'm telling you. I never saw so much blood, except in a maternity case once."

"What happened?"

"He was way down in the woods and his chain saw broke. Flipped right across his face. I'm not sure if it got his eye." He gestured on his own face, from the angle of his left jaw across to his right temple.

Inside the ambulance a pale, middle-aged man lay quietly. He had thought he was going to bleed to death, he told me. Neither he nor his mates could stop it. It was squirting everywhere. Most of his face was covered with a huge pad, held down by a wide bandage wrapped diagonally around his head. Already, blood was soaking through.

"I used maternity pads," said the driver. "I always keep a box on board. I put four across the cut, the two longways on top of them, and bound them on as tight as I could."

It was only an hour's drive to the hospital, so I told the

driver that he had saved the man's life, that I wouldn't touch anything, and to go on into town. Months later, I remembered that original bandage and put it to good use.

During a clinic one foggy, wet day, I was called to see an old man who had taken a dizzy spell while walking down a very steep hill. He fell down, and rolled over and over several times, finally slamming up against some rocks and knocking himself out. Telling the secretary to send the ambulance after me, I set off. I turned right at the post office and started up the hill, and soon came to the accident site.

The patient was sitting propped up against the rocks, while two women pressed a towel onto his head. The old man and both his attendants were soaking wet, and spattered copiously with blood.

"He's split his head right open! Look at the mess!" cried one of them, seeing me arrive.

I asked them if they lived nearby. They both nodded, indicating the closest two houses. Did they have any sanitary pads? And a good strong bandage, like you use on a sprained ankle? They went in search of these items and I took a peek under the towel. To my relief, only the most superficial layer was "split right open". A gash, fully fifteen centimetres long, ran along one side of his bald head, and was bleeding enthusiastically.

The patient was half-conscious, muttering, "Oh my, oh my," to himself, and trying to push the towel away. As I secured the sanitary pads with an ancient ace bandage, the ambulance arrived and took him off to the hospital.

Sometimes the easiest way to get to a house call is to get the patient to send someone to pick you up. A short, stocky, bow-legged little man, at least seventy years old, came to take me to visit his sister on the other side of the town.

When we got out of the car, he indicated a house some sixty feet away down a steep slope. It was bitterly cold, but the sun shone brightly on the smooth ice covering the slope. The tips of the picket fence peeped up through the snow like green teeth. Behind the house the sea sparkled and danced. The old fellow took my large, heavy house call bag and scampered down to the house, without missing a step. I stifled the temptation to sit down and slide, feeling it was undignified. So I crept down, inch by inch, my heart in my mouth.

The patient's daughter welcomed me, commenting on the "wicked" ice. She went on to tell me how, last time the doctor came, he had slipped flat on his back,, and sailed through the front door feet first. He came to a stop in the hallway after knocking over a small table, sending ornaments flying in all directions. The phone had landed on his head, breaking his glasses. She'd had to phone his wife, she said, and get her to bring over his second pair.

While I examined her mother, the daughter made me a very welcome cup of tea. I was sitting at the table writing a prescription, and sipping my tea, when a ginger kitten came up to me, and sat down on the prescription pad. Gently I tried to stroke him with one hand and wiggle the pad out from under him with the other.

Suddenly, he leapt onto my shoulder, and started jumping about and growling. The daughter extricated him, plus a chunk of fur from my parka hood. When she put him down he continued to wrestle with it, growling all the time.

"He thinks it's alive!" exclaimed the patient.

The daughter finally got it off him, but it was in shreds. She was most upset at the damage, but I assured her that it was an old parka. Actually, it didn't show very much.

The patient's brother picked up my bag and ran back up the hill to the car. I followed more slowly. It was less terrifying than going down.

Another way to avoid getting lost is to have someone meet you at a gas station, or other obvious landmark, and follow them to the house. For this call, the turnoff was in the middle of nowhere, and the sign had blown down in a gale. When I got there the only person in sight was a very small boy, with a very small bicycle. As I pulled up he smiled shyly.

"You'se the doctor woman?" he asked.

"Yes, have you come to meet me?"

He nodded.

"Do you want to put your bike in the car and ride down with me?"

"Ooh, yes!"

I opened the hatch and shoved the bike in with my bag and other bits of junk.

"It's me poppy," he explained, referring to his grandfather. "His back's some bad; he can't hardly move. At St. Clare's they cut one of his legs off," he added conversationally.

"Oh, why did they do that?"

"It was ROTTEN," he said, wrinkling his nose at the memory of it.

The road wound around, up and downhill (mostly down) for about five kilometres.

"Did you come all this way on your bike?" I asked him.

"Well, I walked some of the hills, 'cos it was too hard."

"It's a long way for you."

"I'm seven," he said, slightly indignantly.

At the house I went in to see his grandfather, a delightful, friendly old man. I asked if he had seen me before.

"No, and I can't see you now. I've been blind this five years."

It was six months since his amputation, so I asked him if he had his prosthesis. But he had refused one, thinking it would be too difficult to get used to. I told him it would not be as hard as the crutches and would probably help his back. He said he would think about, and he was pretty good for ninety-one, wasn't he? I agreed heartily, and he went on to tell me how the British Army had turned him down in 1914 because he had a bad heart. The doctor told him he wouldn't live to see Christmas.

"Bet that doctor's been dead for years," he said with a chuckle, "and me still here!"

I was almost back to the main road, when I was surprised to hear a deep throaty "Meow!" A large black and white cat appeared from the back seat, and climbed onto my lap. I turned the car and went back, with the cat purring away like a motorboat. When I let it out it ran straight into the house. I backed out and headed for the next call. This one should be easy — I had been there before.

It's How We Say It

The office was busy that dreary spring afternoon. The wind rattled the windows, and it had snowed intermittently all day. Patients came and went, leaving little puddles of water in front of the chairs in the waiting room, from the snow melting off their boots. Periodically, one of the secretaries went round with a mop. On just such a day, a few months earlier, an elderly lady in the waiting room had fallen and broken her hip. She was very nice about it, but it was embarrassing for us. Diane, my secretary, brought in a chart.

"Last one," she said. "Come in Mrs. White."

A fat, middle-aged woman waddled in and sat down. Glancing at her chart quickly, I saw that her last visit had been two years earlier, with a sprained ankle.

"What's the problem?" I asked.

She hesitated a moment or two, then in a rush, "Well, I finds me side, and I feels right logy all the time."

My heart sank. This would take a while to sort out, and could be anything from ovulation to carcinoma.

"How long for?"

"Oh, my dear, since years."

"All the time, or just now and then?"

"At first it was just a scattered time, but now it's steady."

"Does it ever get really bad?"

"Sometimes, it's a wonderful hard pain, and I'm in misery."

"Does it make you throw up?"

"Sometimes I urges with it."

"How about your bowels?"

"Last week I had the scutters, but then, I'd taken opening medicine."

"So you had been constipated then?"

"Yes, but I been like that all me life. Has to take opening medicine, sometimes."

"No change in your bowels then? No blood with it?"

"Oh, no, nothing like that."

"How do you sleep at night?"

She looked surprised. "In me bed."

Trying not to laugh, I tried again. "Does the pain keep you awake?"

"Oh, no. Seems like I get it in the daytime, mostly."

"Have you had a baby recently?"

"No, my baby's eight year old. No, that's not true. His aunt 'ad 'e, and we took 'im. Last one I had meself, well she's twelve year old now."

"How about when you have sex? Do you get the pain then?"

"Well, I 'aven't 'ad any for a while. Me man's in Toronto gettin' 'is stamps."

While she was undressing I considered the possibilities. Here was a forty-five-year-old woman, obviously not neurotic, with lower abdominal pain, fairly severe at times, slight malaise, chronic constipation, but nothing to point to a specific system. I examined her, finding nothing abnormal. I sent her for routine blood work and urinalysis, booked her for a pelvic ultrasound, and told her to return when these were done.

As soon as she had left, Diane entered bearing a mug of tea. Welcome though it was, I groaned. At 5:15 it had to mean she was placating me before giving me bad news.

"Tell me the worst," I begged, accepting the tea, "There's

two house calls to do, each thirty kilometres away, but in opposite directions?"

She laughed. "Not that bad. They just called from the fish plant. They had a boat come in with a seaman they want you to see. I told them to send him up right away. He should be here any minute."

"What's wrong with him, do you know?"

"His hand. He had a rising finger and they took him to the bay hospital at St. Lawrence, where they lanced an apse. So they want it checked, but they sail first thing in the morning."

While waiting for the seaman to show, and my tea to cool, I assembled peroxide, dressings, scissors etc on my desk. The tubegauze applicator seemed to have disappeared, but I eventually located it under a chair in one of the other offices. As I returned to my own office the squeak of the door, followed by thumping footsteps, told me that the (hopefully) last patient had arrived.

"Hello, sir," Diane greeted him, "You come up from the fishplant?"

"Yes, ma'am, this the clinic?"

"Yes. Have you been here before?"

"No, girl, I don't belong around here. I'm from Bonavista Bay. You want to see my MCP card?"

"Yes, please. Is this Workers' Compensation?"

"No, I don't guess. I never hurt meself. It come up on its own."

She took down his information and brought him in. A large young man in wet oilskins and big, heavy rubber boots, he smelled strongly of fish.

"Sorry for the state I'm in, but they said for me to come up right away, as you was wanting to go 'ome."

"That's fine. What happened to your finger?"

"Nothing. It come up by itself. They lanced it at St. Lawrence, and said for me to get it checked in two days. But we was at sea, so it's three days."

As I went to take off the sodden finger stall, covering an equally wet dressing, he flinched. So I asked him if it was really painful.

"I be's afraid," he said sheepishly. "It's not too bad now, but I'm sooky, I guess."

"Men always are," I told him cheerfully. "The women, now, are much tougher. This bandage is in an awful mess! Has it been on for three days?"

"No, the skipper put a new one on yesterday with stuff from his doctor box. It's hard to keep it clean on the boat. Look, I got some waterpups, too."

He showed me the small swellings around his wrists. They look like blisters, but are actually solid, and are caused by the chafing of the oilskin cuffs in the salt water. Having finally got down to his finger, I found it surprisingly clean, and healing well.

"That looks good," I told him.

He examined it doubtfully. "You going to put a new machine on it? It'd be easier to work without."

Telling him to try and keep it clean and dry, I gave him a handful of bandaids, and let him go.

"Doctor box is a new expression to me," I said to Diane, as we put on our coats and boots, "I suppose it's a first-aid kit?"

"Yes, they don't have much in them. Few bandages, aspirin and stuff like that. I think I take more when I go to camp with the Brownies, than they got way out to sea."

Driving home along the slushy roads, I reflected on the expressions Newfoundlanders use to describe their ailments. They are often colourful, especially when combined with the local variations on English grammar, and the dropping aitches off one word to add to another. The dialect made for interesting conversation. Earlier patients that afternoon had complained of a rattle on the chest, an inability to glutch (swallow), and a fierce pain in the back. One patient, previously seen with a puzzling rash, was "best kind" now, which was gratifying, though I still didn't know what his rash was.

I wondered about Mrs. White, hoping she did not have anything nasty. "Finding" one's side, back or whatever indicated discomfort rather than pain. She was clearly anxious and probably thinking the worst. Maybe that was why she felt "logy" — a very useful word, meaning vague malaise or misery. As always the expression "his (or her) aunt had he (or she)" amused me. It referred to an illegitimate child of a relative, usually the sister of one of the couple who "took" the baby. No secret was made of it, and the child grew up knowing who its real mother was.

The young fisherman, who had had his apse (abscess) lanced at a bay, or cottage, hospital, had cheerfully admitted to being sooky, or chickenhearted. But he had worked on, despite what must initially have been a very painful finger, even with a "machine" on it.

The word machine covers every conceivable contraption or gadget. It is also used when the appropriate word escapes one, instead of thingamajig. The request to "pass me a machine" can mean anything from a syringe in an emergency, to a knife, fork, or teabag in the cafeteria.

As Newfoundlanders have become more exposed to — some would say polluted by — Canadian and American culture, particularly TV, some of these unique words are falling into disuse. This is a pity. Even a cursory skim through the *Dictionary of Newfoundland English* reveals many curious and delightful phrases. A man with impotence will complain of "losing his nature" and request a "scrip" or prescription for it. Some patients prefer "medicine" to pills. Even nowadays a patient will want you to "haul" a jaw tooth for him, and be quite put out to be referred to the dentist. "Old Dr. So-and-So used to do it," they tell you, referring to the 1920s. "Only charged a dollar, too."

Many of the old remedies are still remembered, if not much used any more. Most stand-bys for flu, colds, coughs and intestinal upsets primarily contained molasses or alcohol. Snow from the first snowfall in May was collected and melted. It was called maywater, and was supposed to be good for the complexion and sore eyes.

Not surprisingly, many of the old terms relate to childbirth. The baby would be "borned" by the "granny" or local midwife. Soon after the delivery, the neighbours would all crowd in, to partake of the previously prepared "groaning" cake. Ten days later was "upsitting" day, when the mother would receive visitors and show off the baby while sitting up in bed.

A woman box, however, was not a childbirth kit, but a "machine" made to fit on a sled, to transport a sick or injured person.

Death, too, had its own phrases, mostly related to forerunners and premonitions. The dead cart, or death wagon, was the man- or horse-drawn hearse. During epidemics, when people died more quickly than coffins could be made, the dead cart would rumble around the community, picking up the bodies. Death was usually referred to as trouble. "They've had a lot of trouble" meant there had been deaths in the family. "Sorry to hear about your trouble" indicates sympathy for a bereavement.

In the old days, the terms "doctor" and "wizard" were synonymous, meaning any male person — with or without a medical degree — who could cure illnesses, charm warts or relieve toothache. Nowadays, except for charming away warts, most people consult the trained professionals. Whether the results are better is unproven.

Doctor as Vet

Late one evening the nurse on duty came into the staff sitting room.

"There's a fellow downstairs in the clinic," she reported, "He's got his husky with him. It's been at a porcupine, and has quills stuck in its face."

"Eh?!"

"That's what he said. He wants you to take them out. It has to be done quickly, or a reaction sets in. Then you can't get them out, he says."

Much puzzled I went down to investigate. A smiling Inuit stood there, with his dog on a rope. The dog had a dozen quills in his face, and looked most peculiar.

"He can't eat or drink like that. Nothing. You fix him?" pleaded the young man, still smiling.

"I'll try. What do I have to do?" No sense pretending I knew!

"You get thing out of there," pointing at the instrument dish, "and hold quill and pull it out. You have to twist it like this." He gestured with his hand to show me.

The dog was whining and looked quite fierce. Unfortunately my boss, a local man, was away, so I couldn't ask his advice. Nothing for it then, but to do as the patient, or rather his owner, suggested. My reluctance must have been obvious, for he hastened to reassure me.

"I hold him. He not hurt you."

Poking around the instrument dish, I found a pair of artery forceps and, with some trepidation, approached the dog. His owner made him sit down, put his arm around him and held his head with both hands. With the forceps I grabbed the nearest quill, twisted it as directed, and it came out easily. In no time they were all done.

"Thank you. Thank you. He be OK, now." Beaming broadly, he picked up the rope end and led the dog out of the clinic.

That was thirty years ago, soon after I arrived in Labrador, and it was my first experience acting as vet. Unfortunately, most of my subsequent veterinary calls were sad, involving putting down, or pronouncing dead, a much-loved pet.

I don't mind swatting the occasional fly but, really, I'd much rather not be involved in killing animals. The phone rang just as I put lunch on the table. It was Norman. His scruffy, almost tumbledown garage kept most of the local vehicles on the road. More than once I had driven around for a day or two in his battered pickup while my own, much newer, compact underwent emergency surgery. Usually down to earth and sensible, Norman sounded really upset.

"Doc! There's something wrong with Tweedledee! He's took real bad. I think he's dying!"

Tweedledee was one of two identical cats that lived comfortably among the oilcans and spare tires. The other, obviously, was called Tweedledum. Both were plain dirty white, the same size, and had the same face. One morning the previous winter, Norman started a car he had admitted overnight. Out leaped Tweedledum, minus two-thirds of his tail! He wasn't bothered one bit, but it took Norman all morning to fix the car! After that it was easier, to put it mildly, to tell the two brothers apart. Very friendly, they were well-known to Norman's customers. I asked what was wrong with Tweedledee.

"He's having a seizure! Was doing it when I came inside,

just now. He's twitching all over, and his mouth is bleeding. He looks some bad, I'm telling you!"

I went over, of course. Tweedledum was clearly in extremis. Severe convulsions were racking his whole body, his tongue was bitten to pieces, and his eyes were almost out of his head. No wonder Norman was distraught!

"Norman, I can't do anything for him. You'll have to put him down."

"I can't! You do it."

The big man turned his back on me (and Tweedledee) and covered his face with his hands. I took pity on him.

"OK, give me something to whack him on the head with. That will be easiest."

He passed me a wrench that weighed at least twice as much as the cat, and went outside looking wretched. I gave Tweedledee a gentle tap on the head. A revolting squish told it had achieved its purpose. While I was wiping Tweedledee's brains off the wrench with a filthy rag, Norman reappeared, close to tears. He handed me a grocery bag, and we put the cat into it.

"Tonight, after dark, I'll go down the government wharf and drop him in the water. It's good and deep there," said Norman.

"Tip him out of the bag when you do, Norman, so that ... well, so that nobody will see him then."

"OK. Thanks very much, Doc."

A GP friend was left with an unusual souvenir after performing this service for one of his regular patients. He was doing his clinic one morning several years ago, when an old lady marched in. She plonked a birdcage down on the desk in front of him.

"He's old, and logy all the time. Won't eat either," she said.

He stared at her in astonishment. "But I don't know anything about birds!"

"You put him down for me, gentle like. Don't hurt him." She sniffed a couple of times and ran from the room.

The bright yellow budgerigar did look rather dejected, chirping to himself half-heartedly, as he shuffled on his perch. Going through his house call bag, my friend found some Demerol and drew up a vial. He opened the cage and grabbed the bird gently. It didn't resist, and he plunged the needle in where he thought its heart was, killing it instantly. After telling me this sad little tale, my friend looked at me thoughtfully.

"You know, I must still have that damn cage. She never came back for it, and she's dead herself now, poor old thing."

He led me down the basement stairs and opened a cupboard. There, hidden between a defunct vacuum cleaner and an ancient floor lamp, was the cage. He wrestled it out and placed it on the floor.

"It might as well go to the Scouts' rummage sale," he said, and carried it upstairs, where he gave it to his surprised secretary.

People are often more grateful for what you try to do for their animals, than they are for their children. The old and the very young become particularly attached to their pets.

Another GP friend, Olga, who was a newcomer not only to very rural Newfoundland, but to Canada as well, was called one night by an elderly couple about their dog. He had thrown up several times that evening, was "full of gas" and "looked real sick." Olga drove eight kilometres through the blowing snow to the house.

Joey was indeed very sick, hardly stirring as she examined him. His belly was blown up like a balloon, and there were no bowel sounds. Deciding that he had an obstruction, she questioned them about their pet's bowels. They had no idea when he last "went" as he was outside most of the time. Normally he had no trouble, and had been well until three hours earlier.

Unsure what to do, she called a vet in St. John's, 300

kilometres away, and ran the whole story by him. He agreed with her diagnosis and suggested, as an emergency measure, she deflate the bowel with a large-bore needle. If the dog was still alive in the morning, he would be glad to see him, if they could bring him into town.

Olga carried out the recommended treatment — and practically asphyxiated them all! After a few minutes, Joey perked up and looked around. His delighted owners gave him a dish of water and thanked Olga profusely. She tried, in vain, to tell them the recovery might be temporary, and returned home, wondering if she had done the right thing. Next morning, she called them anxiously. Joey was dead, but she had been so kind.

The following week she noticed they both had appointments at the clinic. Feeling embarrassed about the dog, and wondering if they thought she'd killed him, she awaited them nervously. When she had dealt with their medical problems, the old lady produced a package from her bag.

"That's for you, dear, for what you did for our Joey. It was real kind of you."

Now even more embarrassed, she opened the package. It was a warm and cosy pair of handmade slippers, which she wore all winter.

One Saturday I had been on-call and busy with flus and minor injuries. At 7:00 P.M. the clinic was empty at last; then the phone rang.

"Is that the doctor?" The voice was very young, and obviously close to tears.

"Yes, what's the matter?"

"I ... I don't know what to do."

Had she been raped? I wondered. Was she pregnant? Or had she failed her exams?

"What's happened?" I asked.

"M ... my boyfriend was putting away his fishing gear and my kitten jumped at it. Now she's got a fishhook caught in her mouth."

"Who's got a fishhook caught in her mouth?"

"My kitten."

"Did you call the vet?"

"Yes. He's got a recording on saying to call the vet in Gander. I did, and he's got a recording on to say call the vet here!"

"You'd better bring the kitten over to the clinic, and I'll see what I can do. How soon can you be here?"

"About ten minutes. We'll be right there."

Twenty minutes later a motor bike pulled into the parking lot. The two riders were completely in black, from helmets to boots. The passenger held a cardboard box tied up with string.

"Sorry we were so long," apologised Mark, removing his helmet, "It took us a few minutes to catch Fluffy and box her up."

He gently took the box from Heather so that she could remove her helmet. Then we all trooped into the examining room. When I had shut both doors they opened the box, revealing a beautiful grey and white kitten, four or five months old. A length of black thread hung from the corner of her mouth.

"I think it's inside her cheek," said Heather. "I managed to get a quick look when it first happened."

Fluffy stood up, stretched and stepped daintily out onto the examining table. Then she jumped down onto the floor and hid under the instrument table. Heather scooped her up and brought her over to me. I stroked the kitten gently, and talked quietly to her for a few minutes. She lay calmly in Heather's arms, and even purred a little.

But as soon as I tried to open her mouth she became a miniature tiger. Hissing, she wriggled out of Heather's arms onto her shoulder, turned and hissed at me again. No way could I deal with this alone!

What could we do? The nearest vet was in St. John's, almost 300 dark, cold, windy kilometres away. Both the other doctors in the community were gone for the weekend. Then I remembered that a surgeon from St. John's often visited his elderly mother here on weekends. While Heather and Mark soothed Fluffy I went to the phone.

"Lloyd! This is Chris at the clinic. I've got a kitten here, with a fishhook caught inside her cheek. Can you help me?"

"How old is the kid?"

"It's not a kid. It's a kitten, about four or five months old, I guess."

"You mean it's a C-A-T?"

"YES."

"Isn't there a vet here?"

"He's away. So's the vet in Gander. It means a trip to St. John's for them, if we can't help."

"That kitten's going to need an anaesthetic, you know. They're going to have to go to St. John's, Chris."

Returning to the examining room I told the young couple the news. They cheerfully agreed to make the tedious trip. I called a vet I knew in St. John's. He suggested I give Heather and Mark his number, and tell them to call him when they arrived in the city.

"Do you think Fluffy will be OK in that little box?" asked Mark.

It was rather flimsy, and too small to add a blanket. Leaving Heather with Fluffy, Mark and I went down to the basement. There were no suitable boxes, but I found a defunct sterilizer the right size. Wrapped in a towel from the linen, Fluffy looked cosy and snug. She was very calm, and watched the proceedings with interest. The catch on the lid was broken off, but Mark produced a long chain, with a substantial padlock, out of his pocket.

"It's for my bike when I'm at school," he explained.

He wound the chain loosely round the sterilizer and padlocked it, inserting the padlock under the lid to keep it open half an inch, so that Fluffy could breathe. With Heather cradling the sterilizer in her arms they roared off into the night.

Fishhook accidents are commonest in those most-curious creatures -cats - but can, and do, happen to other species. A dog was taken to an isolated cottage hospital with a fishhook caught in its upper lip. The doctor there, a newly arrived CFA (come from away) wanted to talk to a vet before she tackled it. Eventually she tracked one down, and left a message on his answering machine. Over an hour later he called her back, collect, and basically told her to push it through, same as for a human. He advised against sedation or anaesthesia.

The dog, by this time, was thoroughly upset, and it took four people to hold him down. As soon as he felt the hook being pushed through his lip, he began to pee and shit copiously. The procedure was soon done and they released him. The room was a disaster area, with a filthy, slippery floor, and stinking muck on everything and everybody. The dog ran around in circles for a few minutes, thus distributing it still further. Finally, it threw up on its owner's shoes, then crawled into a previously clean corner and went to sleep.

Personally, I haven't been called upon to treat a large animal, which is just as well, as I am rather afraid of them. You wouldn't catch me crawling into a soggy ditch, to attend to a cow with a dislocated knee! One doctor who did was unable to help the poor beast, and the farmer had to shoot it. This happened years ago, when there was no vet in the community.

Quite recently, a colleague received a call from an older woman, a patient he hadn't seen for years. Her horse couldn't make his water, she said, hadn't been able to all day. He was about to tell her to take him to Emergency, when he realized she'd said "horse" not "husband".

"Did you call the vet?"

"Yes, he said give him lots of water and he'd be better in the morning. He said it was because he worked all day yesterday, after doing nothing all week."

"Well, I'm sure that's all right. He knows more about horses than I do."

"But he's just a young feller!"

"Yes, I know, but he's smart. He knows his business."

"You wouldn't know any old Irish remedies, or anything like that, would you?"

"No, girl, I'm sure your horse will be OK. If he's not better in the morning, give the vet another call."

"Well, all right, if you think that's OK."

Very rarely is one called to minister to a wild animal. A public health nurse, working up north, was called one day by the local wildlife officer. He had a polar bear cub, apparently abandoned by its mother, with a nasty cut on its shoulder. Could she stitch it up, please?

After being assured he would tranquilize the cub, and she would be perfectly safe, she agreed and went over to the wildlife office, with a suitable kit. The animal was very young, and its skin comparatively thin and soft. So she was able to put in six sutures, through all layers without difficulty. The cut healed beautifully, and the bear went to live in Edmonton — at the zoo.

As roads and transportation improve, and vets become more numerous, veterinary calls to human doctors are becoming rare. No doubt the animals are as glad as the doctors.

A Vicious Attack

We all see government-funded medical care exploited and abused regularly, by both patients and doctors. It comes as a shock to see what can happen to a sick person without it.

Julian B. was brought to the Emergency Department from one of our city's first class hotels. The housekeeping staff had found him in his room, delirious and very ill. They alerted the management, who called the ambulance. As Julian was wheeled in, lying face down on the stretcher, the attendant commented that he cried out in pain if they tried to turn him over, and that he was "all bandaged up" around his left shoulder. Moving him onto a bed proved both these points, but did not rouse him enough to give us any information.

The hotel gave us his name and home address (which was in England) and said that he was with one of the major oil companies. Apparently, the clerk who checked him in the night before thought he "didn't look well at all." From his time of arrival they assumed he had come off the flight from Boston.

He tried to resist being undressed and examined, but the pain in his shoulder deterred him. The only findings on examination were a temperature of 41°C, a high pulse and low blood pressure, delirium, and a large, messy, stinking dressing covering his left shoulder, neck and upper back. We gave him two suppositories, one aspirin and one acetamino-phen, sponged him down, and turned on the fan.

Then we tackled the revolting dressing, gingerly remov-ing layers of gauze, one at a time. His left shoulder and upper back were mangled, with several deep gouges running across the area. A very deep laceration, close to the neck, had the trapezius muscle exposed. The whole area was oozing bloody, nauseating pus. The surgeon on-call believed the patient had been mauled by a bear. Swabs and blood were taken, an intravenous set up, and a bed in I.C.U. requested. Mean-while, the suppositories were taking effect; his temperature came down to 39°C, and he became conscious.

After confirming his name and giving us his date of birth, he told us he had been attacked by a big dog in Boston. The hospital, he said, refused to treat him, because he had no money on him. After this effort he drifted off again.

For a week his septicaemia threatened to overcome him. His father came over from England, and we learned that Julian was a deep-sea diver, under contract to a multinational oil company. After leaving England, he visited friends in the U.S. before coming to this assignment. The oil company confirmed all this, and made a point of informing the hospi-tal that they were not responsible for the bill, as the present contract had not been signed yet. They said he had not kept his appointment with them, which was at about the same time as Julian had arrived at our Emergency Department. They did, however pay his airfare and his hotel bill.

As Julian's condition improved, he was able to recall some details of the incident. The friends he visited had dropped him off at Boston Airport. Discovering his flight was delayed, he put his overnight bag in a locker and went for a walk. He unwittingly trespassed on private property, and the owner set his dog on him, probably a Doberman. Julian had no idea how he got to the hospital, but the doctor there told him he would only get what he paid for. All he had in his pocket was $20. They took that, applied his dressings and sent him away, despite his insistence that he had insurance and credit cards in the locker. A sympathetic security guard gave him a ride to the airport, where he had just enough time to collect his bag and catch his flight. By the time he arrived at the hotel he was feeling terrible, but put it down to exhaustion and blood loss.

His career was ruined by the incident. His accessory nerve was torn, and his trapezius badly damaged, rendering his left shoulder almost useless. He paid our hospital bills promptly. The oil company demanded he refund them his airfare and hotel bills - as he had not fulfilled his contract. His recovery, medical and financial, was slow.

After this anecdote was first published I had a most interesting phone call from the Scientific Editor of the Boston Globe. He was shocked by the story, and wanted to follow it up. Did I know the name of the hospital where the patient was refused treatment? Could I, without intruding on confidentiality, put him in touch with the patient? I explained that I couldn't remember the patient's real name, and that the episode had happened several years earlier. The newsman then realized that "the trail was cold" and abandoned the project.

After we hung up, it occurred to me to wonder that a small Canadian medical journal would be read in such prestigious circles.

It's a Disaster!

Recently, one of the Newfoundland hospitals where I worked held a disaster exercise. The purpose of these events, apart from being necessary to maintain accreditation, is to test the response of the hospital to the invasion of a large number of casualties. The time taken to locate extra staff at all levels is noted, as are the responses of the ambulance services, police and the fire department. The ability of the mall or school to evacuate everyone quickly is also tested.

One of the objectives, I gather, is the education of casualty officers, usually new grads and/or recent immigrants. Of our four casualty officers, all fairly experienced, two were in St. John's on a course, one was on holiday, and the fourth was thirty kilometres away doing a clinic for a sick G.P. I was relieving, and I've been around long enough to be involved in many disasters, real and imaginary. Personally, I'm hopeless at playacting, and find the mock disasters rather a bore. Real patients are apt to be overlooked.

This one was supposed to be a surprise, but we all knew about it. All morning, spare moments were spent checking supplies and making up charts for the "victims." This was when we discovered we didn't have back-up carts anymore, and hastily threw together supplies for the waiting room and lobby.

At our last mock disaster a year or so earlier, an elderly man had collapsed with chest pain ten kilometres away.

Getting hold of the ambulance crew and explaining they had to go in the opposite direction, fast, was a real hassle. The driver lost several valuable minutes coming to the hospital, and dropping off two "victims" already on board, before answering the call. The patient reached us alive, but soon arrested. Trying to run a real "Code Nine" in the midst of all the confusion was a nightmare, since most personnel thought it was all part of the disaster exercise. Despite our efforts, the old fellow died.

Suddenly, the disaster was announced. Our nursing supervisor got everyone organized and to their appointed posts. She turned to me.

"Chris, you send one doctor out front to triage, one to the lobby, one to the waiting area, and get another one in here."

As the only other doctor in sight was our gynaecologist, I was a bit non-plussed. When I asked him where he would like to go, he stared at me in astonishment. He was just passing through on his way to the caseroom! Our senior surgeon and our senior anaesthetist were both away moose hunting, but the remaining surgeon and anaesthetist both came promptly. They were dispatched, one to triage and the other to the lobby, until their special skills were required. As the first casualties arrived, so did several G.P.s called in from their clinics.

Supposedly, the propane tank at a nearby nursing home had exploded. High school students were co-opted to act as patients. Realistically made up, they entered fully into the spirit of the thing and were really excellent. Interestingly, none of the staff at this nursing home was hurt in the "explosion," and all were available to attend the "victims".

For an hour or so we went full tilt, pretending to assess, treat and document all sorts of desperate injuries in unknown people who were identified only by a tag number. Meanwhile, in the waiting room and lobby, the less seriously hurt were tended and consoled. As we stood back to wait for the lab and X-ray to process everybody, we were told it was over.

We were relieved. No real emergencies had happened while it was going on, and none of the volunteers had been hurt. The year before, one of the kids somehow got a sliver of glass in her neck. it was easily removed, but could have been nasty.

One year, they had insisted that all casualty officers be available. One lived eighty kilometres away, but obediently came in, telling the hospital she would be at my place. After lunch we settled down to play Scrabble. By 3:30 nobody had called, so we called them. The disaster was over and they had forgotten all about us!

The disaster exercise ends at the point when the work is only beginning in a real disaster. In a genuine disaster, decisions must made regarding transfer of the more seriously hurt patients to a larger centre, who should go to the O.R. first, and so on. Anxious relatives, never a factor in exercises, have to see their loved ones, talk to the staff, and be comforted if necessary. Bodies and patients have to be properly identified, and the news media dealt with.

These mock disasters can be disasters in themselves. All kinds of ridiculous mishaps can occur, leading to a total fiasco. Years ago, when I was a casualty officer in a major city, we had a joint mock disaster with the larger hospital across town. A fellow casualty officer and I were designated to go to the scene. When the big day came it would normally have been a day off for both of us, but we reported to the hospital at 9:00 A.M. as directed. After we sat around for more than two hours, the disaster was called.

The police were supposed to transport us to the site of the "accident," a plane crash just outside the city. So they did. In a paddywagon! My colleague and I, and two nurses (both from administration) climbed into the back, and off we went. There were no seats and nothing to hold onto, except each other. As we tore through the city, siren and lights going, we swung around corners, and made sudden stops and starts, with much tire-screeching just like on TV. We were flung about in constant danger of serious injury. Rather scared, we lay on the floor in a row facing the front, and tried to hang on to the floorboards. Suddenly, the driver shouted for one of us to open the passenger side window for him. We looked up to see smoke billowing from the dash. The radio was on fire!

Amazingly, we all arrived at the scene in one piece and set to work. Police and nonmedical people had somehow contrived to arrive first and were rushing busily about, looking very dedicated and important. The team from the other hospital arrived immediately after us, followed closely by the ambulances. We had already been informed that one of the doctors from the other hospital was in charge, and we were to do as he told us. At his direction, we started walking, in pouring rain, to the furthest corner of the field. Halfway across an ambulance came by and gave us a ride the rest of the way.

The scene was utter confusion as supposedly unconscious, or even dead people tried to shelter from the rain, their faces ghoulish , as their makeup ran. Somehow, we assessed everybody in our area, about two-thirds of the total casualties, while the doctor-in-charge directed operations. He was a middle-aged Brit, unknown to me, and had clearly been in the army before going to medical school. Despite the distance and the lashing rain, his voice floated across the field to us. The ambulance drivers, knowing us but not knowing him, kept returning to us for orders, instead of him. The helicopter could not operate due to the rain and poor visibility.

A couple of hours later there were only a few of us left, the staff and some casualties with minor injuries. One was a quiet young man who worked in the housekeeping department at our hospital. He, supposedly, had a broken arm and burns,and was sitting in the field in the rain, cracking jokes with a "corpse" waiting to be taken away. Unexpectedly, he fell back and started a grand mal seizure. We pretended to treat him, but he went on convulsing madly. After more or less ignoring him for a while, it crossed my mind that this could be a real seizure. Maybe he was an epileptic! I suggested this to my colleague, who thought for a moment, then leaned over him.

"George! Next time you and I are on the same shift, I'll make you pay for this!"

The seizure ended dramatically, and George started laughing. By now, however, one of the lay assistants had brought his jeep over. He insisted on getting George onto a stretcher and taking him to the main hospital, as a serious head injury! He also insisted that I accompany him.

As it would get me out of the rain, I weakly agreed and climbed in beside the "patient." There was already one "patient" on a stretcher in the jeep, so I had to half-sit, half-lie between them on the stretcher poles. Extremely uncomfortable, to put it mildly! Seeing this, George sat up, I crawled in behind him, and we were driven to the hospital sitting back to back. once there I followed the signs to the recovery room, handed him over and left. I was somewhere in the depths of the hospital, soaked to the skin, tired out and completely lost. For at least ten minutes I wandered aimlessly about the gloomy corridors, and never saw a soul. Then I came to a window. Looking out, I was able to orientate myself and find my way back to Emergency.

The jeep had long since gone, so I went over to the ambulance garage nearby to get a ride back to the site. The dispatcher told me it was over and to return to my own hospital, five kilometres away. It was still raining. I didn't feel like walking, but I had no money. He couldn't leave, of course, but he called the police for me, and they promised to send a cruiser.

An hour later, still soaked through, and starving, I got back to base to find they were about to start debriefing. My colleague chicken-heartedly slipped into the toilets, leaving me to face a large group of dry, well-fed doctors and staff members. They asked me to give an account of "everything that happened." So I did, leaving out the details of George's "seizure", and just saying I had had to escort a serious head injury to the other hospital.

Most of them had a few laughs, but at the end, a stout, immaculate, middle-aged woman stood up. Later I discovered she was the representative of the hospital board. She imperiously told me that "this sorry tale" was not at all funny, that I looked unprofessional, and might have tidied up and changed before appearing. Furious, I told her that I had only just got back. She pointed out that the exercise had been over for nearly two hours, and where had I been?

Seeing that I was about to explode, the chief of staff intervened, suggesting that the casualty officer who had remained behind give her report. When she was done, this woman criticized her roundly because the "victims" were left in the waiting areas without being seen. It was explained to her, again, that there was a real emergency going on in the department, and that all the G.P.s who were called said they would have come if it was real, but not for an exercise.

A senior nurse reported that the patients who were evacuated from the floors were too ill to spend the whole day in the nurses' residence, being minded by volunteers. Most had not had their lunch or their medications, and were only now going back to the floor.

An hour later, three very tired and frustrated casualty officers met at a diner across the street for a desperately needed meal. My male colleague and I had dried off, and changed into O.R. greens. Our street clothes were ruined. We two women made him pay for the meal, in return for his hiding in the toilet.

The Lighter Side

Work in an emergency department is stressful, hectic, frustrating, demanding and exhausting, but it is worthwhile and never boring. Providing good medical care, in departments which are always too small for the volume of work, and frequently inadequately equipped, is a real challenge. Tragedies are common, but some incidents have their lighter side.

A reporter from the local weekly newspaper could be a real pest. He hung around the Emergency Department when it was busy, ferreting out medical details that were none of his business. It was hard enough to give the patients proper care, let alone privacy, at the best of times. The department was tiny and without doors, except to the undersized resuscitation room. The four curtained cubicles were minute, and not exactly soundproof.

One Sunday afternoon he appeared, very subdued and in considerable pain. His left hand was cradling his right and a ceramic pig. It was his son's piggy bank. Trying to raid it, he had inserted his right baby finger into a hole in the pig's rear end (where real pigs have a hole), turned it upside down, and attempted to push coins out through the slot, by wiggling his finger. Not only was he unsuccessful, but now his finger was stuck!

Rather brutally, I told him that we had two options — smash the pig or cut off his finger. His worried eight-year-old son brightened at the second suggestion. We arranged his hand, and the pig, on the table as comfortably as we could. Taking the heaviest weapon I could find (the plaster shears) I gave the pig a hearty whack. The patient yelled out in pain, but the pig didn't budge.

Our surgeon drifted in and was very much amused.

"You've got a good story for this week's paper, haven't you? Will it get on the front page, do you think?"

The patient glared at him. I offered the shears, but the surgeon went to his office, returning with a heavy paperweight. For several moments he scrutinized the pig, as if deciding where to make his incision.

Then, "OK, everybody, shut your eyes!"

He gave it a sharp smack and pieces of pig flew across the room. Dimes and quarters rolled all over the floor.

"Why did you tell us to shut our eyes?" asked the boy curiously.

"In case you got hurt; those pieces are very sharp and could give you a nasty injury," replied the surgeon. "Be careful as you pick up your money, now. In fact, wait till we've swept up."

By the time the pig was in the garbage, and the youngster had collected all his money, the patient's finger, though swollen and bruised, would obviously recover.

"Thanks," he said humbly, and slunk out the door, followed by his son, with his savings in a plastic bag.

One evening our undertaker, conveniently located next door to the hospital, brought in a man, bent over and clutching his belly, and groaning.

Unable to resist, I said, "One of your customers woke up, did they?"

"No, no, no," he said, shocked. "This is Pierre Duval. He just delivered me a load of new coffins from Quebec. I brought him over, because he clearly isn't at all well. But he doesn't need me yet! Thanks now."

He went back to his funeral home, leaving us to deal with the coffin deliverer, now heaving his guts up in the toilet.

When he subsided we took him to a stretcher, and got him settled down. He gave us his name, address, and medicare number, but his English wasn't up to relating an account of his illness. He was pale and a bit sweaty, but his vital signs were normal, and his abdomen only vaguely tender. Nothing to suggest a specific illness — gall bladder or appendix, for instance.

" 'Ere, doctor, come 'ere," called a voice from one of the other cubicles, "Come 'ere!"

Somewhat reluctantly, I went to this man, very well-known to us. As usual, he was drunk and had been in a fight, and was waiting for me to stitch up a cut on his bald head.

"Them Mounties what brought me in 'ere. One of them's a Frenchie. 'E'll 'elp ye."

I went out to the two officers in the waiting area.

"Either of you speak French?" I asked. One jumped up and came into the Emergency Room with me.

"We've got a fellow here from Quebec with a stomach-ache," I explained, "and he doesn't have enough English to tell me about it."

The Mountie followed me into the cubicle, where the man was lying quietly, but still rubbing his belly. As he saw the Mountie his eyes widened. He sat up, swung his legs over the other side of the stretcher, jumped down and ran out of the department, through the waiting area and out the door.

For a moment we were both too surprised to move. By the time we got to the door he had vanished. Not far away I heard an engine start and a heavy vehicle move away.

Later, the Mountie called me to say that he had run Pierre Duval through the nationwide computer, and even hooked into the QPP network,but had found nothing. Nobody, any-where, was looking for him. Obviously, he had a guilty conscience about something; very likely he was smuggling marijuana, as well as delivering coffins. We never heard any more of him. Presumably, he recovered from his stomach upset and got home safely.

One evening between Christmas and New Year, a very strange figure walked into our Emergency Dept. Clad from head to toe in grey, he was unrecognizable. He strode right up to the desk, where I was writing up a chart, and removed his headgear — an old-fashioned diving helmet borrowed from the museum — revealing himself as one of the G.P.s.

"Why are you dressed up like that?" I asked, staring up at him in astonishment. "Did you think it was Halloween?"

"I'm going jannying," he replied. "This grey tracksuit is supposed to be a suit of armour. I'm St. George."

I asked who was playing the dragon. He named one of the other G.P.s — a very appropriate choice, I thought.

Jannies, or mummers, are a very old tradition, imported from England, where it has almost died out. Though the custom has disappeared in many parts of Newfoundland too, there are some communities where jannying is still an integral part of the Christmas-New Year festivities. Generally, men dress as women and women as men. With mittens on their feet and socks on their hands, a group will go around their neighbours, and dance and sing, and talk in disguised voices, while the household tries to guess who they are. Once recognized the janny has to remove his or her disguise. When all, or most, are identified they dress up again and move on. At any time of year someone speaking strangely, e.g. due to laryngitis, may be accused of "jannytalking."

The G.P. had merely dropped in to ask me to keep an eye on his inpatients while he was gone. He put his helmet back on and went out again, watched with interest by waiting patients.

Some of the experiences I had during my medical career now seem almost as much a part of history as "jannying." Over the last thirty-five years healthcare facilities and telecommunications have developed dramatically, and many of the things I experienced would never happen today. Vastly increased air travel and better roads have made the larger centres accessible to almost everybody, with consequent improvement in living standards and healthcare.